RE-CREATE THE

SENIOR'S
SOUL

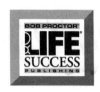

LIFESUCCESS PUBLISHING, LLC
8900 E Pinnacle Peak Road, Suite D240
Scottsdale, AZ 85255
Telephone: 800.473.7134
Fax: 480.661.1014
E-mail: admin@lifesuccesspublishing.com

ISBN: 978-1-59930-179-2

Cover : Fiona Dempsey & LifeSuccess Publishing
Layout: Fiona Dempsey & LifeSuccess Publishing

COMPANIES, ORGANIZATIONS,
INSTITUTIONS, AND INDUSTRY PUBLICATIONS:
Quantity discounts are available on bulk purchases of this book for
reselling, educational purposes, subscription incentives, gifts,
sponsorship, or fundraising. Special books or book excerpts can also
be created to fit specific needs such as private labeling with your logo
on the cover and a message from a VIP printed inside.
FOR MORE INFORMATION PLEASE CONTACT OUR
SPECIAL SALES DEPARTMENT AT
LIFESUCCESS PUBLISHING.
PRINTED IN CANADA

Life is your Journey!
Enjoy, play, live!
Anita Selby

RE-CREATE THE
SENIOR'S SOUL

HELPING YOU ACHIEVE A
HEALTHY LIFESTYLE

ANITA SELBY

BOB PROCTOR
LIFE
SUCCESS
PUBLISHING

TESTIMONIALS

Regardless of age, this book offers insight for everyone in leading a healthy productive life and the tools to help others. We can teach ourselves and others how to prevent isolation, loneliness, and depression and promote health and well-being.

Bob Proctor, bestselling author of
You Were Born Rich

This is a wonderful, readable book that includes work pages and resources to assist seniors in leading a fulfilling life. Highly Recommended!

Gerry Robert, bestselling author of
Millionaire Mindset

Expertly written. Interesting and inspirational. This book will positively impact your ability to age, no matter how old you are. Gracefully educates those who care about aging with the keys to a life of natural wellness.

James "Tad" Geiger MD
The oilMD
Author of
The Sweet Smell of Success: Health and Wealth Secrets

This book is inspirational and thought provoking. It makes us think about what we do in our leisure time and how it impacts our lives. What we think about and how we live our lives has a direct impact on our health and emotional well-being. We need to take time to make a plan that enhances our lives and provides us with an improved lifestyle.

Stacey Grieve, Author of *Why Are You Weighting?*
www.WhyAreYouWeighting.com

Leisure time is no longer about sitting in front of the television; it's about being an active participant in your life. In Re-create the Seniors Soul, *we find out that we are never too old to make something out of our lives. Complete your life, find your purpose, fulfill your dreams..."you are only as old as the people you play with."*

Nancy Ann Lennert, author of
JustAsk.....Let Your Spirit Guide You

This book is a valuable resource! The reader receives important tools as well as insight into how to achieve a healthy and meaningful lifestyle. Well done, a must read!

Lori Humber
Occupational Therapist
Geriatric Assessment and Rehabilitation

TESTIMONIALS

Depression is a world-wide phenomenon, and is not limited to any particular age group. It affects about six million Americans that are over the age of sixty-five, and loneliness can be a contributing factor. Social contacts and increasing recreational and leisure activities are important factors in fighting depression. This book is invaluable in helping us all to discover our interests and our latent abilities, and to utilize our opportunities to improve our health through staying active.

David Butler,
Author of
A "Hand Up", not a "Hand Out"
- The best ways to help others help themselves.

Anita Selby's book Re-create the Senior's Soul *will inspire all of us to take a closer look at how we spend our leisure time. Healthy leisure assists us in improving how we perceive life and manage daily stressors.*

Kim Kapes
Author of From *Wags To Riches*

Our population continues to age and with the knowledge that we receive from a wide variety of media, it is natural to believe that seniors are well taken care of. Unfortunately, there are more seniors becoming socially isolated and are at an increased risk of a variety of problems. Anita's book will help people to set goals that will enable them to lead a healthy life and eliminate the risks of becoming isolated and lonely.

Anita Jackson
Author of **Rekindle the Magic in Your Relationship:
Making Love Work**
and Mediator, Peace Negotiator and Relationship Expert

An excellent resource for the non-pharmaceutical management of depression and provides guidance to living a healthy lifestyle.

Julie Cuthbertson
Pharmacist

TESTIMONIALS

We all seek and receive the benefits of the leisure experience. We may participate in a variety of recreation and leisure pursuits without clearly understanding the benefits we acquire through our chosen activities and lifestyle. As we age, experience loss, experience disease/disorder processes, our ability to participate and receive these benefits can be dramatically impacted. Re-create the Senior's Soul *clearly identifies an understandable approach to overcoming the barriers and challenges that may be experienced in achieving and maintaining a healthy leisure lifestyle. A must read now and for the years to come.*

Kathie Ervin
B.P.A.-Human Services, Rec. T (R)
Instructor Therapeutic Recreation – Gerontology
Lethbridge College

Start early to prepare for the golden years. Even those of us that don't feel like we are quite there yet can benefit from this excellent book. It is never too early, nor is it too late to re-create our soul and prepare for our future. Wonderful insight on how to make the best of and enjoy the years ahead! Anita has written a book that you will find useful not only for yourselves but in assisting your loved ones. Let this book make your life more enjoyable!

Louise Wilson, Videoconference Specialist

PREFACE

After having had three children, I decided that I wanted to go back to school and get an education. I happened to come across this course that was called Therapeutic Recreation, and it intrigued me. One of the prerequisites for entering the program was to interview someone in the profession and write an essay about why I wanted to study this field. The lady that I spoke to had been working with seniors for quite a few years and still enjoyed what she was doing. She was very inspirational, and I found that despite a few reservations, I thought I would love this type of work.

Now, as most people aren't familiar with therapeutic recreation, I will explain it in as few words as possible. Therapeutic recreation utilizes recreation as a tool for therapeutic interventions. There are many different tools for assessment and treatment that are utilized, but I like to say that I use recreation for therapy. Recreation therapists are most often found in long-term care facilities, nursing homes, psychiatry, pediatric wards, and geriatric units in hospitals and also in community settings.

I have been working with seniors for the past nineteen years, and I cannot imagine doing anything that I would enjoy more. The stories and life experiences that seniors share are so interesting. The experiences and often hardships that they have endured, we can only imagine. We live in a world that is filled with conveniences and technology that have made our lives so much easier in many ways. I cannot imagine having to live without a washing machine, dryer, dishwasher, car, or computer, just to name a few of the many, many conveniences we now have. We also live in a time where life moves so fast that we wonder where the week or month has gone. Life seems to pass us by so quickly.

When I listen to the elderly talk about how they used to spend their leisure time, it makes me long for those days. They talk of dances and picnics with neighbors, getting together to play cards or for a quilting bee, or helping one another to build a barn. They were always there for each other, and strong relationships were prevalent in most everything they did. It seems that now we hardly even get a chance to get to know our neighbors. Our lives are so fast-paced that by the end of the week, we are exhausted from everything that we had to do. Weekends are now for catching up on home activities that we are unable to get done during the week. In some ways, it seems life was much simpler then and in other ways, harder. People of older generations worked very hard at everything they did. Men in particular had a very strong work ethic, and if there was not an end product to the activity, it was not worth doing. Farmers especially seemed to hold this philosophy. There were always chores to be done, and they were busy from very early in the morning until the sun went down at night. Family was very important to them, and women, as a rule, were able to stay home and look after the children and home. It is quite a stark difference from the way the normal household looks today.

I believe that I was attracted to this profession, as many things fell into place in order for me to get into my current position. Many doors opened at just the right time, and the right people were put in my path. The Law of Attraction was available to me even though I did not understand the full potential of this wonderful law. In retrospect, I can see very clearly how everything fell into place for me to be in the job that was meant for me.

I recently was motivated to write this book to help seniors and their families create a healthy leisure lifestyle and possibly prevent deterioration in health and mental and emotional well-being. The Law of Attraction can help maintain a feeling of connectedness to the universe and the social supports that we need as we age. Social supports are the most important factor in helping to maintain health and happiness. Isolation is a contributing factor to death among the elderly. Yves Saint Laurent was a millionaire with fame and fortune but no friends. He ultimately died of loneliness. Don't allow this to happen to you or your loved ones. Share this book with friends, family, neighbors. Brainstorm together and make a plan for success. It could change your life!

The future belongs to those who believe in the beauty of their dreams.

—Eleanor Roosevelt

DEDICATION

TO MY HUSBAND STUART. Without your support, this would not have been possible. I appreciate your encouragement and your belief that this book will be beneficial to so many people. Thank you, my love.

To my grandparents and parents, who have taught me that life is a journey and that we all have wonderful things to offer over the course of our life span. Getting older is part of this exhilarating experience we call life, and it is what we make of it.

ACKNOWLEDGMENTS

I would like to thank the seniors that I have had the privilege of working with over the past twenty years. The knowledge and wisdom that you have shared have been valuable in so many ways.

Thank you to the wonderful staff that works on the Geriatric Assessment and Rehabilitation Unit for their support and encouragement over the years. You have imparted untold knowledge and growth in the field of geriatrics and psycho-geriatrics since we initially opened this unit, and the benefits to our community and the health of the seniors have evolved into something to be proud of.

To my children: Shawn and his wife Lindsay, you have the most beautiful family, and your love and blessings have always meant the world to me. Christina and her husband Curtis, thanks for listening to me and letting me share in your life with your family. To Matthew, your struggles will make you a stronger person. I love your wit and intellect.

Embarking on this journey to write a book has been exciting as well as frustrating at times, but the support of my brother Rick and his wife Kelly and my sister Cynthia has never wavered. Thanks so much for believing in me.

To my mom and dad, Toni and Adolf, thanks for always being there for me, including some very trying years. You have always stood by me even though you may not have always agreed with my decisions.

My in-laws, Louise and Dale and Bryan, for letting me be part of your family and encouraging me in my endeavors.

And more than anyone else, to my wonderful husband Stuart who has been my inspiration and support from the very beginning. Thank you for being you.

INTRODUCTION

I have worked as a recreation therapist for the past twenty years in a variety of care settings for seniors. I love working with the elderly population and derive pleasure from hearing their stories and words of wisdom. They have so much to offer in terms of life experience that even after twenty years, I continue to look forward to the life stories of my patients.

The profession of therapeutic recreation is both challenging and rewarding. Recreation therapists work with people of all ages and are dedicated to improving quality of life for those they serve. It is a profession that performs assessments and develops interventions based on individual needs, strengths, and goals. Recreation therapists look at functional abilities in three areas: treatment, leisure education, and recreation participation. Recreation therapists believe that leisure and recreation are integral components of optimal health. For the purpose of this book, I am focusing on teaching seniors to set their own leisure lifestyle goals that will guide them to an improved quality of life.

In order for us to maintain balance in our lives, we need to look at all aspects of our well-being. Many people tend to think that recreation and leisure are not an important component to quality of life. Without time to relax our mind, body, and spirit, we are unable to rejuvenate ourselves. In order to maintain daily functions, we must be capable both mentally and physically. As we age, our free time can become overwhelming, and we are often uncertain as to how to fill our days. As we go through our lives, we tend to fit in the "fun" things when we can and look forward to the day we retire, or when the kids are grown up and gone, or when we can move into a condo, or the various things we need or want to accomplish in our lives. All of a sudden, we get all of those things, and sometimes, all the free time can be overwhelming. Now, how do we fill those long days; what can we do? We may need to adapt our activities to physical limitations as we get older, but there are many ways to overcome barriers.

There is a saying that states whatever we sow, we shall reap. Our attitude has a powerful influence on how we manage life. We choose whether they are negative or positive attitudes; it is entirely up to each individual how you will grow your garden. Let me explain. Whichever attitude you plant into your mind will grow. Imagine two seeds, one being a beautiful rose bush and the other seed poison ivy. Both will grow when you plant them in the ground. And the more attention you give them through feeding them and giving them water and sunshine, the more both will grow. Now our attitudes are like those seeds, and the choice you need to make is whether you feed the negative or the positive attitude. You need to decide what you want growing in your heart and mind.

Getting motivated can be an overwhelming task when one is faced with obstacles and barriers. As we learn to have fun and enjoy our life, our self-esteem and willingness to learn and grow is magnified. We can learn from each other, friends, neighbors, children, sibling, spouses, and acquaintances.

INTRODUCTION

Continue to think positive thoughts, and set some goals. It will help you to focus on what you want to achieve in your life, and when you take the time to write it down and put it in a prominent place, it will provide you the motivation to keep going. This book will take you through the process of setting your own goals and bring you an improved sense of well-being.

TABLE OF CONTENTS

CHAPTER 1

RECREATION AND LEISURE

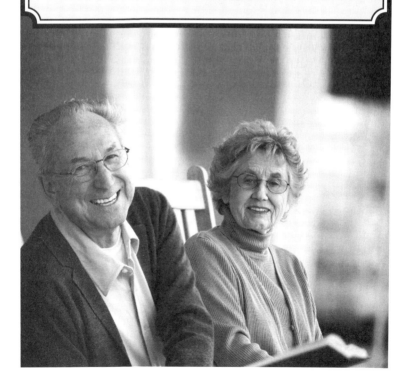

CHAPTER 1

Recreation and Leisure

"Recreation's purpose is not to kill time, but to make life, not to keep a person occupied, but to keep them refreshed; not to offer an escape from life, but to provide a discovery of life."

— **Author Unknown**

Recreation can be defined as the use of time for therapeutic refreshment of the mind, body, and soul. It constitutes active participation in diverting and fulfilling activities. Research has shown that recreation improves quality of life, life satisfaction, and overall health and well-being. Recreation is essential in counteracting stress and can be used as a diversionary tool by people with chronic pain and other health issues. No matter what age you are, recreation is a major factor in maintaining a healthy life. Just think about how boring your life would be if you had no recreational stimulation. How would you fill your day? What would you do besides sit and think about your physical ailments and everything else that may be wrong? Recreation can be a very useful tool in diverting attention from the humdrum or stressful events of everyday life and can help us focus on positive events while putting the stressors in the back of our minds for a little while.

Recreation can help us to fulfill all of our needs in a holistic manner. As mentioned earlier, recreation addresses a person's mind, body, and soul. Though these aspects of a person's overall health are different, they are also related. Psychological health encompasses our emotional and mental health and is instrumental in determining our physical health. People who are psychologically healthy develop awareness of and are in control of their thoughts and feelings, which leads to a healthy, fulfilling, and satisfying life. This awareness has physical benefits because we use our bodies to fulfill the demands of the activity. Whether it is walking, dancing, playing badminton, biking, or any other activity, various parts of the body act to make the activity work. It seems so simple: when we make our bodies work, we exercise that part and improve its functioning. Imagine: we can improve muscle function, flexibility, cardiovascular fitness, and weight control in one activity. What an easy way to keep our bodies fit! We can have fun, be competitive, and get fit all at the same time.

When we make our bodies fit, we feel better about how we look, our minds are sharper, and our self-esteem improves. How we perceive our quality of life improves too, and it feels good. Recreational pursuits make us feel good on a deeper level than the physical. We are stimulated on a cognitive level that can help us improve our ability to think and function more highly.

There is also an inner good feeling that says to us, "Wow! I am excited about what I just did!" Despite feeling exhausted and physically drained, we still feel good.

I do many different recreational activities to make me feel good. In the morning, I run on my treadmill or outside (when the weather is nice). I enjoy going to the gym after work, and I have taken up belly dancing! I do these activities because I like to start my day on a positive note. I feel good physically when I run, and it helps me get my day started with lots of energy. I go to the gym after work to rid myself of the daily stress of my job. I can work those weights and release any pent-up frustrations from the day so that I don't bring them home with me. I like belly dancing because it teaches flexibility, muscle control, muscle memory in learning choreographed dances and moves, and stamina. There are also many social benefits. I attend belly dancing with a friend, and that gives me the opportunity to socialize in a friendly environment.

Leisure is a spiritual and mental pursuit. It is time that is free from other obligations. Some say it is a state of being and can be seen as a form of rest or entertainment. As a rule, leisure activities are restorative and often include activities that are aesthetically pleasing. These are often activities that we do simply for the pure joy of doing them like listening to music or reading a book. Many of us deny that we even have any leisure time. We are so busy performing the functions of daily life that we think there is no free time. Some of our daily tasks may be things that we enjoy doing, and we tend to think of them strictly as tasks that require our attention. For example, I have a little vegetable garden in my backyard, and though it needs my attention to maintain it, I actually enjoy having my feet in the soil and weeding it. The same holds true of my outdoor hanging flowers. It brings me pleasure to tend to them and watch them flourish.

Some of us were brought up to believe that if you had time on your hands, you were not being productive. You needed to fill your time with sewing or crocheting something needed for the household. That is no longer the case. In the past, sewing, cooking, or fixing the car were essential activities because there was no one else to do them for you. Now we sew or bake or tinker on vehicles because it provides us with a sense of pride and accomplishment, not simply because we have to. We can do these things merely for the joy of doing them. They can help pass the time, and we feel good about our final product. Depending on what you enjoy doing, leisure can include baking, making crafts, woodworking, or repairing cars. With leisure activities, we can achieve the good feeling that embodies the mind/soul wellness model. There is such a variety of leisure pursuits available to us that I am sure we hardly recognize them: music, art, reading, playing games, visiting with neighbors, babysitting grandchildren, and the list goes on and on.

> Some of us were brought up to believe that if you had time on your hands, you were not being productive.

I enjoy attending the symphony. It gives me an opportunity to dress up and maybe go out for a nice dinner beforehand. The experience of sitting in the audience and listening to the beautiful music fills my heart with peace and fulfillment.

I marvel at the abilities of the musicians and the conductor and the dedication required to perform at such a high level. I appreciate the work that has gone into the performance and enjoy listening to the music. The whole experience is rewarding to me because it fills my soul and restores my mind.

I WOULD LIKE TO MAKE A DISTINCTION BETWEEN RECREATION AND LEISURE.

LEISURE CONSISTS OF relatively self-determined activity-experience that falls into one's economically free-time roles, that is seen as leisure by participants, that is psychologically pleasant in anticipation and recollection, that potentially covers the whole range of commitment and intensity, that contains characteristic norms and constraints, and that provides opportunities for recreation, personal growth and service to others. [1]

THE DEFINITION OF RECREATION is: to renew or enliven through the influence of pleasurable surroundings; to refresh after wearying toil or anxiety, usually by change or diversion; the act of recreating or the state of being recreated: refreshment of the strength and spirits after toil; diversion, play; a means of getting diversion or entertainment. [2]

RECREATION CONSISTS OF activities or experiences carried on within leisure, usually chosen voluntarily by the participant—either because of satisfaction, pleasure or creative enrichment derived, or because he or she perceives certain personal or social values to be gained from them. It may also

1. Kaplan, Max. Leisure: Theory and Practice. New York, New York: John Wiley and Sons, Inc. 1975.

2. Webster's Third New International Dictionary.

be perceived as the process of participation or as the emotional state derived from involvement. [3]

Recreation involves a time commitment, especially if you are on a team, while many leisure pursuits can be more individual in nature. If you were on a baseball team, for example, and chose to continuously not show up, your teammates would certainly not be too happy with you; not to mention that you would lose out on the benefits of attending the ball game. The leisurely pursuit of attending an art exhibit does not require your attendance to continue, but again, if you do not attend, you are the one who misses out on the benefits of the activity.

> You need to have leisure time in order to do recreational activities. As mentioned earlier, leisure time is time free from obligations or daily activities.

While the definitions of recreation and leisure differ, there are similarities, and the terms are often used interchangeably. Recreation and leisure are compatible. You need to have leisure time in order to do recreational activities. As mentioned earlier, leisure time is time free from obligations or daily activities. Both recreation and leisure activities promote wellness. While recreation plays a larger role in the physical aspect of well-being, it also involves the mind and soul. Leisure pursuits primarily focus on the mind and soul and, to a lesser degree, the physical aspect. Take, for example, walking. Some people walk for the exercise; they take it very seriously and do

---

3. Kraus, Richard. Recreation and Leisure in Modern Society. Santa Monica, CA: Good Year, 1978.

it regularly. This would be a recreational activity. Others may enjoy going for a walk to see the different sights, stop and look at the flowers, or just to take their dog out for a walk. Here, there is a more leisurely component to the activity of walking. One activity can achieve different goals for different people, and what their expectations of that activity are may change, depending on their needs at that time.

In the past, recreational activities were often seen as an opportunity to visit neighbors or family. It was time that was free of obligations, but there was not as much opportunity. During the early to mid-1900s in America, farms and communities were often very far apart, and neighbors could be miles away. Recreational opportunities were not abundant and took much more planning. Going to a dance was a big deal and a highly anticipated event. These farmers worked very hard on their land and homes and, given the opportunity to get together, would play just as hard. The work ethic was very strong and continued with some people into their senior years. This attitude held especially true for men who needed to produce a product in order for an activity to be of any benefit or value. The attitude was: If there is nothing to show for it, what is the purpose? I still hear this comment, especially from men when I assess their leisure interests.

There has been a shift in attitudes over the later part of the twentieth century, especially with all the new research and studies being done to show that recreational activities produce results beyond a finished product. For example, the act of playing soccer or going to a dance has physical as well as social benefits. This was known instinctively, but the benefits were never fully understood. These activities, and others like them, are now viewed as valuable because they provide diversions that have restorative properties and contribute to general health and well-being. The same value is also held for leisure pursuits. Not too long ago, if you had free time on your hands, the first question was, "Why? Don't you have chores that need to be done or homework that needs attention or something else that is productive?" That was certainly prevalent in my house growing up, where I never had the opportunity to be bored. If I had nothing to do, my parents certainly found something for me to do. Don't get me wrong; I had ample time to play and be a kid, but I learned to never complain about having nothing to do. My parents grew up in a very different era and came from a European background. They had nothing when they came to Canada, and both of their families had to work very hard to get ahead. My father worked in construction as a bricklayer and eventually owned his own company. It certainly was not handed to him; he worked many hours to achieve his goals and provide a stable home for his family. My mother also worked full-time, and both parents tried to secure a good life in which they could enjoy the fruits of their labor. In my parents' era, leisure pursuits were treasured times mostly spent with family and friends. Today, we have far more leisure time than past generations. We have far more conveniences like washing machines, dishwashers, vacuum cleaners, lawn mowers, and computers than our parents or grandparents did. While they spent their time doing tasks that were time consuming but necessary, we can load our dishes in the dishwasher and go do something else. We spend more time in front of the television set and are entertained by other media. As our free time expands or decreases according to where we are in our life cycle, what we do in that time frame also changes.

As we age, our needs change. We progress through life, and our recreational and leisure needs are reflected in what we do. When my children were young, my free time consisted of driving them to soccer, dancing lessons, BMX racing, karate lessons, and whatever activity they happened to be doing at that time. I was a Brownie leader, my husband was a Beaver/Cub leader, and whatever activity the kids were in, we were also involved. We felt that it was important to teach our children the importance of team sports and being active within the community while learning new skills and staying active. They also had their share of time playing video games and playing with friends.

When kids grow up and move away from home, parents' needs change. We have more free time to explore activities and leisure pursuits. The activities that I pursue at this stage of life are more directly related to the things that I like to do or learn. I have the freedom and flexibility to grow as an individual, be creative, and attempt new things. My leisure time has increased dramatically, and even though I am still committed to a work schedule and maintaining a household, there is ample time to explore activities, new or old. It is an exciting time! This is a time for us parents to become more aware of the health benefits of recreation and leisure and pursue them wholeheartedly. We can volunteer our time to various organizations and get more involved in religious organizations or other groups and clubs. Our free time can become more focused to meet our own needs.

Our needs for recreation and leisure increase as we age. Reaching retirement can often be a difficult adjustment for some people because of this. I often dream of the day that I can retire and not have commitments that require me to get out of bed and be somewhere every day. But I have had people tell me that retirement is not all that it is cracked up to be. We dream of it for years, and when the time finally arrives, we really don't know what to do next. All of a sudden we have far more free time than we can handle. "Now what?" we ask ourselves. "How do we fill our days? How can we be productive and feel like we are still contributing to society?" There are many things that we don't consider when we think of retirement. We have lofty goals but no real plans. I think, "Wouldn't it be nice to travel and volunteer my time as I see fit, yet not really be committed to anything?" In my retirement, I want to have the freedom to come and go as I please, but I have no real goals. When I talk to elderly people, they often tell me that they are bored and sometimes lonely and that they don't know how to fill their days. Housework, yard work, cooking, personal maintenance, and bill paying do not require large amounts of time to finish, leaving ample time to fill. We are more educated in the benefits of quality leisure time than our grandparents were and recognize that we need to have more things to do in order to maintain a high quality of life.

> In my retirement, I want to have the freedom to come and go as I please, but I have no real goals.

As a society, we are now more aware of the benefits of recreation and leisure. There has been a switch in attitude that has created a higher demand for more opportunities for recreation services in communities, nursing homes, senior centers, and even hospitals. The therapeutic benefits of recreation can be useful for every age group—from therapy that uses play to interpret problems in children, to child-life specialists in pediatric settings in hospitals that can use recreation as a diversion to help the children heal faster, to nursing homes where recreation therapists plan programs and activities for residents to promote quality of life and maintain functioning. The programming and assessments being done by recreation specialists and therapists provide their clients with activities to aid in growth and stimulation.

There are many studies being done that look specifically at different therapeutic interventions for all age groups with a variety of barriers or disabilities. These include pet therapy, relaxation therapy, aromatherapy, music therapy, guided imagery, and meditation. The benefits of these interventions have shown significant results in helping clients improve their quality of life. We all know the saying, "Music can calm the savage beast." Well, researchers are proving that there is some merit to that statement. Music provides opportunity for reminiscing and relaxing. Many people in palliative care use music to help them relax. I work in a geriatric assessment and rehabilitation unit, and we provide a music program to the patients at least once a week.

There is also a big push to promote healthy lifestyles as a form of preventive health care. We are being bombarded with information about how to live a more fulfilling and healthy life. Television ads suggest people should get out and walk more, and more studies and articles are being written in a variety of magazines and newspapers that encourage participation in the community. Information about how to engage in a healthy lifestyle is readily available to anyone looking. And it is not just physical activities that are being encouraged. Television ads and research articles also promote healthy diets, discourage smoking, and provide education about the effects of alcohol misuse, to name a few topics. Advertisers and researchers are attempting to provide us with the knowledge that will enable us to think proactively rather than reactively about our own health. I have seen several programs developed that encourage healthy, active living for seniors that discuss everything from fitness to medication use.

There are now more centenarians (people reaching the age of one hundred) than ever before, and the numbers continue to grow. The Boston University School of Medicine performed the New England Centenarian Study, which began in 1994, and their findings suggest that at that time, there were 40,000 centenarians in the United States with 85 percent of them women and 15 percent of them men. Some of the studies conducted and stories written about these remarkable people found that leading a healthy, active lifestyle plays a significant part in aging well. Less stress and more social stimulation, as well as good nutrition, also play a role. Leonard W. Poon, PhD, director of the Georgia Centenarian Study at the University of Georgia in Athens, says his center's studies have shown that centenarians generally have remained active throughout their lives. They also smoked less, drank less, and ate less than other people.

The most surprising research suggests that socialization plays a significant role in living a long life. A sense of belonging and purpose helps keep the mind alert. Centenarians express a high level of satisfaction with life and often play a significant role in the family or community. Centenarians have shown that, generally, they maintain a healthy weight, do not smoke, handle stress well, are able to cope with loss, have a high degree of self-sufficiency, are resourceful, have a great sense of humor, and look forward to the future. They often stay engaged in hobbies, volunteering, and have other interests as well. Some studies that look at successful aging have found that adults over the age of seventy-five identify the following factors as important to aging: family and friends, health and well-being, spirituality, community involvement, and new learning experiences.

Following good health practices will increase the chances of living a life that is free of disabling and chronic diseases.
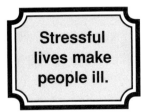
It is never too late to make changes to your lifestyle. Research is now predicting that if you follow good health practices, you can extend your life expectancy. Good health practices include keeping physically active, watching your weight, not smoking, not drinking excessively, getting adequate rest, eating breakfast, and reducing snacking between meals. Social stimulation is also a very important aspect of increasing life expectancy. Those who are socially isolated have a mortality rate that is more than two times as great as those who are socially active.

Stressful lives make people ill. People with stressful lives tend to feel hopeless and helpless. In times of stress, the body secretes the stress hormone called cortisol, which can impair the immune system. Having a sense of control over your life can

---

* Berkman, Lisa F., Breslow, Lester. Health and Ways of Living: The Alameda County Study. New York, New York: Oxford University Press, USA, 1983.

lower stress levels and improve overall health. Taking control of your health and well-being can make you feel that you are the master because you control your destiny and make decisions based on your need for a healthy lifestyle. You are the only one who can truly make those decisions even though you may feel stuck in a situation that you are not in control of.

The first of the baby boomer generation are quickly reaching the age of sixty-five. This generation will have a higher demand for services, including recreational services. There will be an increased demand for social stimulation, for places to meet, for learning skills, and for having a sense of control. This generation will want to make choices about what services they want to participate in and also have a say in the quality of services that are being provided. This generation has learned to fight for what they want, and I believe that is a very good thing. That is what our society believes in, what our laws suggest we should be afforded—the right to demand the services we require. Many senior centers and communities are starting to meet the intellectual, creative, leisure, and health needs of older adults. Many people are starting to understand the holistic perspective of health and well-being. They are looking for opportunities to improve themselves through a variety of means—health, nutrition, mental stimulation, and spiritual connectedness. They can be found in colleges and universities taking courses in karate, tai chi, or meditation and relaxation to improve their health and mental well-being. The possibilities are endless! The stereotype of the aged is changing, and society is accepting the fact that seniors are able-bodied and productive contributors to society. Many seniors work well beyond retirement. It gives them a sense of belonging and of being productive.

Some seniors may retire earlier and decide to pursue other activities. Some may find a part-time job doing something that brings them pleasure and gives them a sense of purpose. Others may volunteer with different organizations or agencies, again, providing them with a sense of purpose without having the feeling of being tied to a job. Others still may just plan to work on their home or travel. These will likely be younger retirees with different interests. Many senior centers are acknowledging the younger retirees (those fifty-five to sixty-five) and providing activities to fit this age group. Local agencies will likely be used more fully as swimming pools, fitness centers, senior citizens centers, and condos are becoming more desirable to this generation. Most condos provide fitness centers and pools, recreational areas to play pool and shuffleboard, and many other social/recreational activities. It also allows them the flexibility to travel and not worry about getting someone to watch their house while they are away.

CHAPTER 2

BENEFITS
OF RECREATION

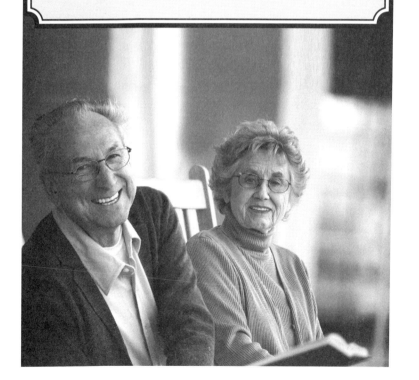

CHAPTER 2

Benefits of Recreation

Recreation enhances our quality of life. This includes a sense of meaning and purpose. What this means is that what we offer, whether it is advice or doing a job, is appreciated and makes us feel like we have provided someone else with something of value. Recreation helps us develop a sense of purpose and can make us feel like we are making a meaningful contribution. This helps us to feel that we have purpose and increases confidence. The mental, emotional, and social benefits include, but are not limited to, a positive self-image, feeling less stressed and happier in general, increased memory and reaction time, and reduced anxiety and depression. Many experience the ability to relax and sleep better and consequently have more opportunities to socialize because they have more energy to go out. Seniors specifically have identified some desirable outcomes such as independence, participation, fairness, dignity, and security.

BENEFITS OF RECREATION

Recreational and leisure activities have the ability to provide us with fulfillment—a sense of elation and joy in having done something that feels good when we complete the task in a satisfying manner. Have you ever done a crossword puzzle? There is a sense of satisfaction in completing the puzzle. I really struggle with crossword puzzles, so when I can complete the whole thing, I feel a real sense of accomplishment. Whether it is a sedentary activity or a very active sport, the feeling of accomplishment and fulfillment permeates the completion of the activity. Why is it so hard, then, to start doing some of the things we enjoy doing? Why do we not long for the elation we receive from an activity seen through to completion? Lack of motivation! We need to find ways to motivate ourselves to get started.

To get motivated, we need to be aware of the positive events in our lives and recognize that we create those same positive events. You can play a role in your own happiness. When you can master both the good and bad events in your life, you are contributing to an overall sense of well-being. Healthy living is more than just the physical aspects of health. It involves a thinking process which affects our bodies, and what we do with our bodies affects how we feel emotionally. I believe that recreational and leisure activities re-create or rejuvenate your mind, body, and soul. Mental well-being implies a capacity to deal with all areas of life, including contentment. To maintain good mental health is to have a positive self-image, be autonomous or self-determined, and have the ability to manage life. Having a sense of direction or goals and a conviction that life is worth living creates a sense of purpose. Being involved or becoming involved in activities can make one feel that life is indeed worth living. Someone who is mentally healthy has no difficulties making new friends, maintaining relationships, and avoiding potentially harmful relationships. In general, people who cope with stressful situations successfully adjust well in later adulthood. They tend to minimize stressful events through positive appraisal and active ways of coping. When you keep your mind stimulated and active, you continue to grow intellectually. When your mind is stimulated, it affects how you feel about yourself in a physical sense. This stimulation can happen on many different levels through different activities. For instance, learning can take place through reading, crafts, sports, dance, meeting new people, and engaging in social activities. Doing things like making puzzles, playing games, writing letters, and reminiscing with others challenges your mind. When you don't use your mind it, like an inactive body, can become sluggish. Many older people feel that happiness and contentment increase with age, but you must keep yourself stimulated!

As we age, our muscles and joints don't do what they did when we were twenty or thirty years old. We can, however, keep them working at the optimal level if we continue to use them. Our bodies deteriorate very rapidly if we don't use them. Recreation provides us a fun way to keep ourselves fit. The more we do, the easier it becomes, and the same holds true if we choose to do very little. The old adage, "If you don't use it, you lose it" holds true. It is far too easy to sit in front of the TV and do very little. Go bowling instead, or take the dog for a walk. Just get active!

Re-creating the soul refers to "feeling good"—a feeling of excitement and contentment, of achievement, of conquering an activity. Feeling good about our achievements means feeling good about life. Re-creating the soul creates a high level of consciousness and exhilaration that comes from an internal place deep within us—an accomplishment that is rejuvenating and stimulating, that makes us feel alive. This can come from volunteering, learning a new sport, being with other people, getting out of a rut, or contributing to society.

When we "feel good," we increase our emotional well-being. This is a benefit of leisure pursuits. When we accomplish a task, we feel a sense of pride; we feel good about ourselves, and we can look at ourselves as contributing to our own lives in a positive way. You should be able to look at yourself in a mirror and feel really good about who is looking back at you —that is an accomplishment! When I go to the gym after work, at the end of the activity I feel like I have released the stresses that I accumulated throughout the day, and I am able to go home and fully enjoy the activities that I do with my family. When I was younger, I used reading as a way of having some peaceful time. It was "my time," and while I was raising three children, it provided me with a break in my day that gave me an opportunity to rejuvenate myself to continue on with the demands of being a mom and a housewife.

> **You are what you believe you are. If you feel like you cannot accomplish a task, well guess what?**

You are what you believe you are. If you feel like you cannot accomplish a task, well guess what? Chances are that you will not be able to perform that task. Henry Ford once said, "Whether you believe that you can, or whether you believe you can't, either way, you are right." This holds true for all aspects of life. Recreation allows us an opportunity to try a variety of activities that we feel comfortable with. If we are successful with them, our self-esteem increases. We can overcome obstacles by being persistent. We do have what it takes to succeed! We can develop our skills, and, when we stick to it, our self-efficacy improves along with our self-esteem. As we develop our skills in one area, we are often more willing to expand our horizons and look for additional learning experiences. We can expand our skills and learning experiences to promote how we think and feel about ourselves. We can begin to feel worthy.

When we feel worthy of interacting with society, we are more willing to extend ourselves. We will take the initiative and look for opportunities that will allow us to feel good about ourselves. There are so many opportunities for us to extend ourselves and provide for others while improving our own feelings of self-worth. Maybe you could go to the local school and talk about your experiences, or maybe you go the library and work with children and read stories. You may feel comfortable assisting in providing social activities in a nursing home for those who do not have many social supports. You may want to teach others a new skill or craft. We tend to believe that we do not have much to offer others. But if you take the time and look at the skills that you do possess, you will be amazed at the abilities you have within you to make a difference in the lives of others as well as yourself. Whether or not you comprehend and accept the emotional benefits of being involved in your community, you intrinsically know that what you offer does have an impact on others. We all need to feel appreciated, and there are many ways to improve how we feel about ourselves and our lives.

Recreation also provides us opportunities to make a positive difference in our physical well-being, which can be measured through a variety of methods. There are tests designed to measure several areas of fitness, from flexibility to cardiovascular levels. Just the act of going for a daily walk can improve your cardiovascular health, improve muscle strength, maintain your weight or help shed unwanted pounds, and decrease the risk of hypertension, colon cancer, and diabetes mellitus. Adding weights can also aid in reducing osteoporosis and decrease the risk of falling by improving muscle strength, coordination, and balance. Proper exercise can maintain and strengthen the muscles and keep us more active for much longer.

Social well-being means being connected to other people and to the community. Being connected to the community creates and maintains a well-rounded social identity which, in turn, creates self-esteem. Maintaining a rich social life feels eventful, active, stimulating, and challenging. Try to be involved in at least one community organization. Some studies have shown that this type of role leads to good health and longevity. Having many friends and acquaintances is also associated with good health and longevity, while having smaller networks can lead to poor mental and physical health. To promote social well-being, it is also important to maintain relationships with family and peers and to have at least one confiding relationship.

I have heard many people say that they are not able to perform certain tasks due to different limitations. Sometimes these limits are self-imposed. I interviewed a woman who said that she was not able to do anything because of the arthritis in her hands and the pain associated with that. Research has found that if she continued to use her arthritic hands, their function would improve and the pain would decrease. The same "use principle" applies to other functions of our bodies such as our cognitive abilities. The less we use our muscles, the more they deteriorate and the less we feel like doing anything. It becomes a cycle. That cycle needs to be broken in order for the body to maintain the ability to carry out the tasks of daily living. The same thing applies to our cognitive abilities. We need to continually use these functions in order for them to perform optimally.

> There is no monetary gain from doing these things; the gain comes from the internal feelings we get from the act of doing and giving.

When we think about spiritual needs, we most likely think about attending church or believing in God or a higher being, but spiritual needs can also relate to the giving of oneself for the greater good of the community. There is no monetary gain from doing these things; the gain comes from the internal feelings we get from the act of doing and giving. Volunteering your time and energy to what you believe in is a good cause and will likely generate psychic income. Psychic income is not measured by monetary gain; it gratifies the psychological and emotional needs such as power, prestige, recognition, and fame. In my community, there is a volunteer association that promotes volunteer placements for the whole community. These can range from a hospital setting to a variety of different agencies and organizations. What a valuable way to spend your free time and achieve your psychic income!

Denis Waitley said, "Time and health are two precious assets that we don't recognize and appreciate until they have been depleted." We never really appreciate what we have until we no longer have it! How many times have you been sitting at home wondering what to do? How many hours do you spend watching TV? Do you wonder how you can spend your time in a more positive and productive manner? If so, you are seeking a sense of spiritual well-being. Look around, and see what resources are available to you. Get involved for your own sake!

Social stimulation is valuable to all human beings. The mortality rate for those who are socially isolated is two times as much as those who are socially active (Berkman and Breslow, 1983). For people over the age of seventy, social isolation significantly increases the risk of death (Kaplan, 1992). When one considers the magnitude of that finding, social stimulation becomes a very important factor in an individual's well-being. Who would ever have thought that keeping to yourself can actually increase the risk of death? Loneliness and lack of companionship or social support can leave the elderly vulnerable to heart problems. A study being done by the University of California has found that among the older adults in the study, for each unit increase in loneliness that was measured, the odds of being diagnosed with a heart condition increased threefold. Some research has suggested that social losses and social isolation appear to weaken the immune system. These are some very good reasons to get active and seek out companionship and new friendships.

In general, I have found that people like to talk about themselves and their experiences. Who do you share your experiences and stories with? Your life experiences have value, and it is important that you share them with others. It is even more rewarding when you find someone who has shared some of those same experiences and can relate on a personal level. I enjoy watching seniors interact with each other. Their experiences differ so much from what my life experiences have been. I often wonder if this generation could survive the events and advances in technology that our senior population did. When I think of the changes in our society over the past seventy to a hundred years, it seems like science fiction from the fifties is no longer science fiction. It makes me wonder what the next hundred years will bring. Just think, in the twentieth century, we went from the horse and buggy to cars, planes, bullet trains, ships that can carry aircraft, and the use of the internet and cell phones. I can still remember when my aunt had a party line on the farm, and she was considered among "the lucky" to have one. Today, the technological advances are tremendous. You can interact with people on the Internet, and many people have used these interactions to build friendships with people from around the world. In some ways, our world has become much smaller, yet in other ways it has become more impersonal. How well do you know your neighbors?

There is comfort in knowing your neighbors—that they watch out for you, and in return, that you watch out for them. The support that we can receive from each other can be tremendous, especially in times of need. I have seen many people whose neighbors have intervened on their behalf, and it has saved lives. Not only can we help ourselves by being socially active, but we can also make a difference in someone else's life. As Jany Wyman put it, "The opportunity for brotherhood presents itself every time you meet a human being."

New learning experiences have value for us as well. We can increase our knowledge base, learn new skills, and increase our repertoire of activities that we participate in. An increasing number of seniors are enrolling in colleges and universities. They are endeavoring to increase their knowledge base and possibly achieve the education they were not able to have earlier. The sense of accomplishment in completing a course brings its own rewards. Chances are, they are not getting this education to get a job or a promotion; they are doing it for the joy and sense of accomplishment that goes with it. Many will also attend recreation and leisure classes to expand their knowledge base in a more recreational atmosphere. These classes provide an opportunity for socializing, making new friendships, keeping the mind active, providing stimulus, and giving a sense of purpose, which all contribute to feelings of self-worth.

Relaxation through leisurely pursuits can allow us to feel rejuvenated. If we take time to read a book, meditate, or listen to nice, relaxing music, we give ourselves time to get away from the troubles and worries of daily life. Allowing ourselves to be peaceful and participate in an activity that we enjoy in a calm and sedentary way relaxes not only our brain, but our body as well. Again, we are able to cope with life in a manner that is peaceful.

When we are able to release our anxieties and stress, we allow ourselves to heal emotionally or feel better on an emotional, and sometimes spiritual, level. Emotional health is the ability to understand feelings and achieve emotional balance, while spiritual health is the sense of who you are, your purpose for living, and that innermost part of your being that allows you to gain strength and hope. It allows you to discover and develop a sense of meaning in your life. When we can free ourselves from pent-up anger and frustrations, we open ourselves up to feeling better about our day. Then we can focus on what is ahead of us in a more refreshed manner.

When we can release all that baggage, we will find that our ability to concentrate and focus improves. Our mind is no longer muddled with all the bad stuff that happened during the day. We can concentrate and look forward to the rest of our day or evening. Our ability to shed that weight from our shoulders can lead us to a more productive and healthy relationship with others.

When we can get through all of that, we find that our self-worth improves as well. As has been mentioned before, when we have a stronger belief in our self-worth, we have more energy, and with more energy we can redirect our energy outside of ourselves by helping other people. When we are focused on how we can help others and not on what they can do for us, we can improve our own self-esteem by feeling that what we have to contribute is of value to others.

When you become detached mentally from yourself and concentrate on helping other people with their difficulties, you will be able to cope with your own more effectively. Somehow, the act of self-giving is a personal power-releasing factor.

—Norman Vincent Peale

GETTING INVOLVED IN activities helps us combat boredom and loneliness. When we are active in any type of leisure or recreational pursuit, it gives us a sense of purpose, a reason for waking up each morning, and we feel good about starting a new day.

Leisure and recreational pursuits help us to fill our need for recognition. We all want to feel like we are needed, to feel that we belong to a group or society as a whole. We all want to know that what we are doing can benefit ourselves and others.

A patient that I worked with recently is now ninety-two years old, his wife is ninety-one, and they are still living in their own home. He hired help for the yard work, and they get help with the house work as well. He is very proud of the fact that he continued to golf until he was into his nineties. He doesn't look like he is over ninety years old; in fact, he looks like he could be in his seventies, at most. He continues to be full of life and has an incredible sense of humor. He is an inspiration to many around him and carries a positive personality and zest for life.

To laugh often and love much; to win the respect of intelligent persons and the affection of children, to earn the approbation of honest critics; to appreciate beauty; to give of one's self, to leave the world a bit better, whether by a healthy child, a garden patch or a redeemed social condition; to have played and laughed with enthusiasm and sung with exultation; to know even one life has breathed easier because you have lived--that is to have succeeded.

—Ralph Waldo Emerson

CHAPTER 3
LEISURE CAN HELP US COPE WITH LOSS

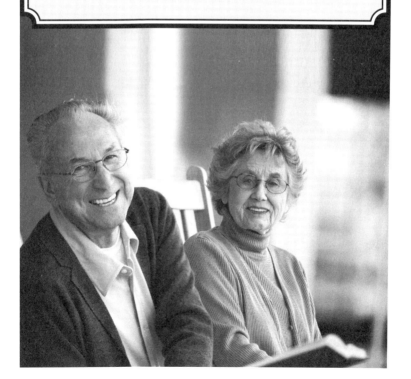

CHAPTER 3

Leisure Can Help Us Cope
with Loss

As we get older, we experience more losses of those who are dear to us. When we experience a loss, we go through a grieving process. Dr. Elisabeth Kubler-Ross has identified five stages in the grieving process. The first stage deals with denial and isolation. We deny that the loss has taken place and may withdraw from social contacts. The second stage is anger. We feel anger toward the person who died for inflicting pain on us, or we feel anger at the world for allowing the death to happen, or we feel anger at ourselves for allowing the death to happen, even if there was nothing that could have been done to prevent it. The third stage is bargaining. We believe that we can make a bargain with God to bring that person back to us. The fourth stage is depression. The fifth stage is acceptance. Finally, we accept the reality that our loved one is no longer with us. During the whole process, it is common to have many conflicting feelings, including sadness, shame, anxiety, loneliness, and guilt. Experiencing all of these feelings can be very stressful. If you look after yourself well, grief can pass more quickly. It helps to have a close circle of friends or family. It is important to eat a healthy, balanced diet, drink enough fluids, and get lots of exercise and rest.

Support groups can be a very useful tool for helping us deal with loss. If you are experiencing difficulties with accepting the loss of a loved one, there are counselors that deal specifically with grief. They are well equipped to help you work through the process and get you to the other side where you can feel whole and healthy again. There are wonderful support groups in some communities, often offered through the local senior center or religious organizations.

Support from family and friends is very important. When someone dies, it seems like there is a lot of support initially. Then, over a period of time, all the support seems to fade away. During this time, don't be afraid to ask for help from your family. If you don't ask, they will likely never know if you need help. It is very helpful to be around others and reminisce about your loved one. Wonderful memories are a useful tool in overcoming grief.

Remember that you are not alone in this. Use your social supports which help you keep in touch with the world around you and keep you from slipping into depression. Use the resources around you, despite the fact that you think you can do it on your own.

Social supports are healthy to lean on in times of grief. Family members are valuable, as they tend to gather around and help work through the grieving process. This process is not cut and dry; many people go back and forth between the various stages. If family members are aware of these stages, they can help everyone cope with the loss. When we understand that we do not all grieve in the same way or in the same time frame, we allow more flexibility for everyone to grieve in a healthy environment. Some people might just say, "Hey, pull up your socks and get on with life." Maybe some people can do that, but that is certainly not how everyone deals with grief. Many of us are left with a void in our lives, and that is a difficult obstacle to overcome. For example, when you have been married to someone for over fifty years, and you are used to doing things together with other couples, it is difficult to socialize with those couples now that you are single. It is vitally important to let people help you.

> Grieving is a difficult process that takes a lot of energy out of us.

Friends also become a valuable asset when we are grieving. Social outings or having friends over helps provide us with stimulation and an outlet. Friends not only offer their support, but just their presence can also be a comfort. Again, the social stimulation of being with others has value and benefit. Even though we are grieving, and we feel like the world around us has crumbled, social and recreational activities can help divert us and help us focus on ourselves in a healthy manner. Our friends often try very hard to get us motivated to move on with our lives. This is difficult to do when you have lost someone who has been a very meaningful part of your life. But do let go and let your friends help you. That is what they truly want to be able to do.

If we are religious, places of worship may become a very important part of the grieving process. Our spiritual being looks to God or one's definition of a higher being for guidance and acceptance. We need to know that our loved one is okay and that we are going to be healed. We seek council through the words of the Bible. This can bring comfort to some. A spiritual community can offer activities, functions may take on a new meaning for some, and it is a wonderful place to be with other people. Whether it is God or some other spiritual energy that you believe in, our universe will heal if we allow it to.

The most common way people give up their power is by thinking they don't have any.

—Alice Walker

I HAVE TOUCHED on the idea that diversional activities can be beneficial when we are mourning. When we divert our attention to another activity, it takes our mind away from the pain. It allows us time to reflect, as well as to rejuvenate ourselves. Grieving is a difficult process that takes a lot of energy out of us. We need to find ways to increase our energy levels so that we can move on and be an active part of society again.

I spoke to one woman who said that when she was grieving, she did a lot of walking. She went to the malls and found different walking paths in the area she lived in. She felt that walking was not only a good way for her to reflect on life but also gave her an outlet for her frustrations. Walking, or other strenuous activities, allows us to work out our frustrations, pain, or even guilt. It is very difficult to motivate ourselves when we are in so much pain. I can't stress enough how important it is to get out and be active.

Sharing memories of your loved one is a wonderful way to remember them. There are times when we find out things about someone only when they are no longer with us. When my grandmother passed away and I was reading her obituary, I discovered that she wrote poetry. In fact, she had some of her poetry printed in Germany. This was something that I had never known about my grandmother. What a pity I wasn't able to share that with her.

I was talking with a young woman who had lost her husband in an accident. She said that in the year since her husband died, she learned more about herself than she could have imagined. She felt that as an individual, she learned just how strong and independent she really was. She was learning to fill new roles and was experiencing life in a whole new way. Though she and her husband had a very strong relationship, she is still able to find her new life exciting. The way that she has dealt with the loss inspires me. She has grown through the experience and has a positive outlook on her life.

Pets can be very therapeutic at any time, but when your life seems empty, a pet can provide needed companionship. I am a dog person and have a little bichon. She is so entertaining and loveable. I did not want to have a dog in my life. I felt that because my children were grown up and gone, I should seize the opportunity to travel whenever I wanted. My husband really wanted to have another dog. I eventually relented, and we got her. She has become very much a part of our lives. She even jogs with me on the treadmill in the mornings.

One of the physiological benefits of having a pet includes the ability to relax. For example, watching fish can be very calming; it decreases heart rate and blood pressure. Some people even feel a spiritual fulfillment when they are with their pets. Another benefit is the involvement of touch. For some people, touch from another person may not be acceptable, yet touch from a dog or cat is very therapeutic. We become more empathetic when we are around animals, perhaps because what you see is what you get. In human interactions, we are not as direct. We can also develop an outward focus when we deal with animals. There is the ability to be in an emotionally safe environment that is nonthreatening and nonjudgmental. Animals accept you without qualification; they don't care how you look; they are uncomplicated and forgiving. Even people who do not like animals often enjoy their antics.

Having a pet can also help decrease feelings of isolation or loneliness. Caring for a pet can give us back a sense of purpose because we are caring for and nurturing another creature. For many of us, our pet becomes part of our family unit. Sometimes our pet gives us a purpose, like when we have to get outside and take the dog for a walk. Pets certainly have the ability to fill a void in our lives.

Relaxation therapy and techniques can also help us cope with loss and stress. Given the right conditions, relaxation therapy and techniques give the mind and body the chance to do their own healing, restore harmony, and help create conditions for optimum living. They allow us to release both mental and physical tensions. For relaxation therapy, a significant range of techniques are used, some of which go back thousands of years, while others are still being developed. They are all based on the effect that the mind has on the body. Relaxation therapy provides a nonintrusive, gentle approach to help treat a variety of ailments such as arthritis, depression, high and low blood pressure, and stress-related mental and physical problems such as panic attacks. There are lots of ways to learn relaxation techniques. Your local library or book store likely carries both books and CDs on how to use relaxation therapy.

Aromatherapy has also been gaining ground as a holistic treatment for caring for the body. As an alternative medicine, it is one of the fastest-growing industries, though it has been around for six thousand years or more. Hippocrates used aromatherapy in baths and scented massage. Today, botanical oils can be added to the bath, massaged into the skin, or diffused into the air. Aromatherapy can also be used to alleviate pain, care for the skin, and invigorate the entire body. When inhaled, it works on the brain and nervous systems. The essential oils that are used come from plants, flowers, trees, fruits, seeds, grasses, and bark. They have distinctive qualities which can improve and prevent illnesses through psychological, physiological, and therapeutic properties.

Aromatherapy uses essential oils to stimulate the sense of smell. We have the ability to distinguish over ten thousand different smells. These smells enter the limbic system, which is the part of the brain that controls our moods. There is lots of information on aromatherapy, and which aromas work best for what ailments can be found on the Internet as well as many books specific to aromatherapy. There is far too much information to discuss here, but I did find a wonderful Website called Tranquilities for Persons Experiencing Grief. Bob Miller, ND, is one of the creators of this program which uses aromatherapy, guided imagery, sounds, music therapy, and your personal religious faith to help you through the grieving process. (The Website will be listed under resources in the back of the book.)

Guided imagery is also a very useful tool in the process of healing. It has been used for centuries and is now becoming used as a powerful tool for stress management and coping strategies. It is a mind-body intervention that is aimed at easing stress and promoting a sense of peace during difficult times. It uses the power of the mind to assist the body in the healing process and involves all five senses to balance the mind, body, and spirit. It can reduce muscle tension and promotes relaxation using imagery that triggers the unconscious and stimulates positive emotions. It can help to cope with lifestyle changes and also be an avenue to identify and communicate one's inner feelings when dealing with stressful or difficult times. It provides opportunities for people to focus on positive thoughts and images. Some research has shown that guided imagery can reduce stress and anxiety, decrease pain, reduce side effects, decrease blood pressure, help with diabetes by lowering blood glucose levels, reduce the severity of headaches, and enhance sleep, self-confidence, and quality of life.

Listening to music can also alleviate stress and has always been a great healer. In the Bible, David played the harp to ease King Saul's severe depression. Music is a mood changer and can work on many levels at the same time. The rhythm of the music has a calming effect, even though we many not be conscious of this. In later stages of life, we respond to music by associating it with the safe, relaxing, protective environment provided by our mother's womb. The body's energetic system is influenced by sounds. The physical body responds to certain tones and frequencies, so when we choose the right music, it will help to put us in a state of calm.

Music brings back memories for most of us. I can relate certain songs to specific times in my life. I have watched people listen to songs that can make them cry or bring very happy memories of childhood. War songs, for example, can elicit many different emotions for people—some very strong and some very meaningful. Listening to music can be soothing to people who are anxious or agitated if you select the right kinds of music. I have watched a local harpist work with individuals who are agitated and upset, and she is able to calm them with her musical talents on her harp. I have seen music used for relaxation. I have known people who won't participate in other activities, but will come out of their rooms to listen to music. Music is a nonthreatening activity that can stimulate social interaction but can also eliminate the need to socialize with others if the individual is not yet ready for that.

Music has the ability to change your mood. When I am sad, I tend to listen to sad songs. What I should be doing is listening to songs that will change that mood into making me feel happy. Sometimes, the music we listen to can reflect what we feel. If we are aware of how the music is affecting us, we can move into changing what we are listening to in an attempt to change the mood and emotion we are feeling. When I exercise,

I don't listen to sad music; I listen to music that is upbeat and stimulates the flow of energy. When I clean my house, I like to listen to music that I heard as a kid when we had to clean the house. This has a dual purpose: it brings back childhood memories and encourages me to get my house clean. Music can be a very influential part of the healing process. Find out what works for you. Experiment with different kinds of music, and take note of how it makes you feel. Then allow it to take you where you want to go.

Meditating is also a practice that can help us cope with loss. There are many types of meditation, but a generally accepted definition is, "consciously directing your attention to alter your state of consciousness." Traditionally, meditation was used for spiritual growth to become more aware of a guiding presence in life. Recently, meditation has become popularized as a valuable tool for finding peace, relaxing, and relieving stress. Meditation can also be used for healing, emotional cleansing, increasing concentration, manifesting change, developing intuition, and finding inner guidance and creativity.

> **Meditating is also a practice that can help us cope with loss.**

Some meditation techniques that are used include rhythmic breathing, deep breathing, visualized breathing, progressive muscle relaxation, music-assisted relaxation, and guided imagery. Once again, if you look at your public library or local bookstore, there are likely a variety of books and CDs available to teach you how to meditate.

Proper nutrition is often neglected, especially when we are going through the grieving process. As we age, changes in lifestyle can affect our eating, but when we are grieving, eating is one of the last things we think about. The thought of cooking can be overwhelming, especially when you have lots of people around. Order in if you have to, but proper nutrition can make a difference in how quickly you recover. When we eat properly, we can increase our mental acuteness, increase resistance to illness and disease, and have higher levels of energy. Eating right can help us maintain a positive outlook on life.

Once you are on your way to healing, you may want to adjust how you prepare food. Cook enough for a few meals and freeze some of it. That might help to carry you through those days when you just don't feel like cooking. At least you will have a nourishing meal that doesn't require much fuss. You may want to join a cooking club or have potluck evenings with neighbors or friends. This will provide you with the opportunity for social stimulation as well as access to good nutrition. The other thing you could consider is cooking larger amounts and sharing with a friend or neighbor. Have your family over for Sunday dinner. When you are focused on preparing a meal for others, you are again diverting your attention and focus away from your grief. Socializing with others can help you to move on with life.

If you're a senior, attending the local senior center is a good way to get out and make new friends, learn new skills, and get active. It can be difficult to make that initial step, but most senior centers have lots of different activities for you to participate in. Most have support groups, provide meals (at extra cost), and offer a variety of social opportunities. It is frightening to start to venture out and try new things, especially if you are now alone, but you may find that there is too much free time on your hands, and going to a center can help to fill a void. You may find that you will connect with other people who have similar interests. Our local senior center has travel opportunities. They plan the trips and calculate the costs. Some find this easier than trying to plan a trip by themselves. Plus, it provides comfort to know that someone familiar is going on the trip, and that you are not left out there all on your own. I also know people who travel totally on their own and love every minute of it. They feel that they are not responsible for anyone else besides themselves and are free to do whatever they want, whenever they want. We all have different expectations and needs in life. We need to identify them, plan with those needs in mind, and move forward. Either way, a senior center can help keep you active and provide you with the people and activities to refresh your mind and body.

There are many different activities, organizations, and supports that can be undertaken to help cope with loss. We need to make a conscious effort to use them, especially when we are hurting from losses in life. Being with other people will ease some of the burden of the pain and help us move on with our lives. I dealt with a woman who had lost her husband the previous year. She was a retired school teacher who loved working with younger children. She started doing some volunteer work through the local public library with children and young students who were learning how to speak English. She was very excited about working with kids and found a purpose in life again.

All men and women are born, live suffer and die; what distinguishes us one from another is our dreams, whether they be dreams about worldly or unworldly things, and what we do to make them come about... We do not choose to be born. We do not choose our parents. We do not choose our historical epoch, the country of our birth, or the immediate circumstances of our upbringing. We do not, most of us, choose to die; nor do we choose the time and conditions of our death. But within this realm of choicelessness, we do choose how we live.

—Joseph Epstein

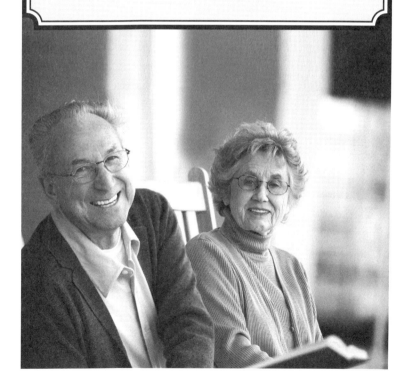

CHAPTER 4

SOCIAL ISOLATION CAN KILL!

CHAPTER 4

Social Isolation can Kill!

Social isolation is a lack of contact, interaction, or companionship with others and causes feelings of loneliness. However, loneliness can be experienced even in the presence of others, and some people can live alone without being socially isolated or feeling lonely. These are the people who tend to participate in activities outside of the home or have significant numbers of visitors or home supports. Living alone, however, is a major factor in the potential for social isolation.

Some of the causes of social isolation can be living alone, health problems, loss of roles, widowhood, and lack of finances. The loss of roles can include things like retiring or changing from the role of a spouse to that of a caregiver. Declining health and other physical limitations can also lead to isolation and put people at higher risk for social isolation. As the elderly tend to not want to intrude by asking family members to take them in or look after them, living alone is becoming more prevalent in our society. Many wish to hold on to their homes and the memories that are in the home. It is difficult to release that independence, and this can often lead to living at risk in the community. Poverty or lack of financial stability may come to those who suffer most from social isolation. The aging baby boom population is projected to have an even higher rate of social isolation due to decreased rates of marriages, higher divorce rates, and fewer children.

Research indicates that social support is a human necessity. Those who are socially isolated are at an increased risk of mental illness, physical decline, and even death. Social isolation is a gradual yet complex process that is often associated with seniors and advanced aging. It can start by not wanting to go out and participate in things that we had always enjoyed doing. We may slowly find that getting groceries is a real chore, and we choose to have them delivered. We may quit going to church or visiting with friends and family. Over a period of time, we find we are not doing anything at all. Our day is spent watching TV and tidying up the house. Just the thought of going out becomes overwhelming.

When we start to feel like there is no one to talk to or confide in, we need to look at what we are doing and make a concerted effort to increase our social contacts. Even if you start with just a phone call to a friend, you need to reach out and maintain those contacts. Often we may not even recognize that we have isolated ourselves. Do you feel lonely or bored? What do you do when you feel this way? Do you feel powerless? Are you filled with self-doubt? Do you feel confined or deserted? Are you having difficulty setting goals for yourself? Do you have trouble making decisions? These could be symptoms of social isolation.

I often see people who have become socially isolated. Sometimes it is because they have lost a spouse or because their physical health is starting to deteriorate; sometimes they are no longer able to drive. When we begin to explore the barriers that lead to social isolation and what options are available to combat them, we can begin to open doors and start to make a difference. There are many opportunities for socializing with others; sometimes we just need to know where they are and how to access them. Talk to others who are active or your health care providers, or go to the phone book and look for listings of different agencies and organizations in your community. There are likely more services in your community than you know of.

Sometimes people use visits to their doctors as an opportunity for a visit or social stimulation. This can have some real negative effects. When you are sitting at home all day, all your aches and pains seem to intensify. You go to the doctor to try to ease it, and before you know it, you are taking far too many medications for ailments that may or may not be real. Many seniors take far too many medications. Look in your medicine cabinet. How many bottles of prescription medications do you have there? If you are not using them, take them to your pharmacy and have them disposed of properly. Take note of what your pharmacist says about mixing medications. There can be some pretty dire consequences from some medication interactions. Be smart and look after your health.

Some people will also use alcohol as a way to escape. It is especially dangerous to mix this with medications, as alcohol reacts negatively with over one hundred fifty different medications. When medication and alcohol are combined, it puts you at risk!

Alcoholism in the elderly is more prevalent than most of us realize. It is estimated that over three million seniors in America have some type of alcohol abuse disorder. The highest rate is found in widowers over the age of seventy-five. A study was done on suicides that looked specifically at people over the age of sixty-five, and the results showed that 35 percent of men and 18 percent of women suffered from alcohol abuse.

When you don't get out of the house, you will decline physically. Your muscles will not get used enough, and they will deteriorate. This becomes cyclical. When you start to lose your ability to mobilize or you tire easily from exertion, you don't feel like doing anything,

> **Maintaining old friendships may be a good place to start.**

and your physical decline escalates. Do you see how this can become a downward spiral? You have to fight this right from the moment you see it happening. Do not allow yourself to become a statistic!

Maintaining old friendships may be a good place to start. Research has shown that over half of the people who are in their eighties still have one close friend. The most common sources of new friendships for the elderly come from community associations, like churches and senior centers. Men are more likely to make friends through associations while women tend to make friends in their neighborhoods. Long-standing relationships promote well-being better than new friendships. Sometimes even a phone call to a close friend can invoke that feeling of well-being and connectedness. We all need some form of intimacy, and friendships can provide some of that for us.

Sometimes writing letters back and forth to friends who no longer live close by gives us a sense of belonging. We can confide in close friends even though they may not be physically close. The Internet is a wonderful tool for being able to stay in contact with people. Many community colleges and senior centers have courses on how to use the computer and how to access the internet and chat areas to help you stay connected with family and friends. No, you are not too old to learn!

Loneliness can be combated by having a sense of control over some aspect of your environment. Remember that you choose what you do with your life and how you make adaptations for your deficits. You do have control over what you do and how you do it. It helps to have someone to confide in, to let someone know how you feel and what some of your difficulties are. Maybe they can give you suggestions to get you out and more active. On the other hand, maybe it is you who can help a neighbor get out and be active.

Stroke survivors are at high risk for becoming socially isolated. When they first experience a stroke, they are so focused on regaining whatever deficits the stroke left them with. They are anxious to get better so they can go home. Leisure interests are usually not a concern at the time of rehabilitation, but it does become a real issue after they get home. All of a sudden, they are left with some deficits, and they are no longer able to perform the tasks and activities that they used to. Recreation therapists are very good at helping people overcome and adapt to their deficits, but not everyone has that luxury. Stroke support groups are very helpful in dealing with all the struggles associated with strokes. Many places also provide support groups for the caregiver and/or spouse. We often forget that a stroke not only affects the person who had the stroke, but it also affects the caregivers and the people around them. What used to be routine is no longer possible. Many adjustments need to be made. Leisure activities need to be maintained in order to prevent social isolation of both the victim and the caregiver. Talking with other people who have gone through this experience is a good resource. It is important to realize that you are not the only one out there who is experiencing the things you are going through. Check with your local hospital or senior center to see if they are running support groups or if they are aware of any in your area.

It is important to maintain social contacts as well as you can. You need to access the support systems in your community. There are opportunities in larger centers for day programs and respite care, and rehabilitation centers or clinics often assist in the recovery process. Accessing services like Handi-bus to get you around when you can no longer drive is very helpful. Losing the ability to drive is a big loss; it takes away your independence, and you need to rely on others. That's what services like Handi-bus are for. Utilizing these services helps to overcome the barriers to enjoying your life. Set yourself goals. Start with small ones, and as each day progresses, continue to set higher goals for yourself.

Alzheimer's disease and other forms of dementia seem to promote social isolation. In the early to middle stages of the disease, people often recognize that they are starting to be forgetful and don't want to put themselves in a position that allows others to see their deficits. It is important to remember that both mental and social stimulation is very important to maintain. I worked with an individual who was in the mid to late stages of Alzheimer's disease. Both he and his wife would play Scrabble together every day. She believed that it was important to keep his mind stimulated for as long as possible and felt that it was beneficial. She was right. There are now medications available to help slow down the disease process as well. In the later stages of the disease process, attention span becomes very short, and it is difficult for the patient to attend to most activities for any length of time. It is helpful if you can find familiar tasks for them to perform to keep them occupied and stimulated. It could be washing dishes, sweeping the floor, or sanding pieces of wood. It needs to be something that is familiar to them and that they have a good understanding of how to perform. Music is a very useful tool as well. I have watched people who are not able to perform simple tasks continue to play the piano or sing the words of a complete song. When I discussed this with one of the geriatricians, I was told that music is stored in a different part of the brain and is not affected by Alzheimer's until the end stages. I found it absolutely incredible that they could retrieve entire songs but not be able to focus enough to put a sentence together.

Again, in many communities there are support groups for Alzheimer's patients as well as for the caregivers. The Alzheimer's Society may be a good place to start. Often, it is the caregivers who need the most support in how to handle some of the behaviors of the affected individual. There may be respite care services available, day programs specifically for Alzheimer's sufferers, and emotional support from home care workers and providers. We are not able to manage this care all by ourselves, so ask for help. We tend to think we can manage everything on our own, but then both patient and caregiver become very isolated. Caregivers need to carry on with activities outside of the home so they can manage day-to-day care-giving needs. Maybe you can count on a family member so you can go out for coffee or to a movie with a friend. We need to take the time to rejuvenate ourselves so we can continue with the demands that are placed on us. I see so many caregivers who are burned-out with the responsibility of caring for their loved one. That includes both spouses and children. They are trying so hard to keep their loved one in their own home for as long as possible that they often become ill themselves and then are no longer able to provide care.

Parkinson's disease is another process that can initiate social isolation. Many people with Parkinson's do not want to be seen by others, especially if their tremor is very noticeable. People with Parkinson's disease need to maintain an exercise program that includes aerobics, as well as strengthening and stretching activities. This is so important for maintaining mobility, flexibility, range of motion, and balance. Loss of range of motion in the joints or tightness in the muscles can aggravate the symptoms of Parkinson's, leading to increased difficulty walking and performing daily tasks. Exercise can also help relieve depression and constipation.

Support groups can be very helpful for many people, as they provide education, support, and advice for people living with Parkinson's disease. Support groups also provide opportunities to meet other people who have similar experiences and can be a source of practical information about living with the disease. To keep you from getting socially isolated, you may want to look to your church or other spiritual community as a way of getting involved in different activities. This will help with your spiritual development as well as stimulate social interaction with others. You can develop some very good friendships and support systems through different church activities. Many of the larger centers offer activities through senior citizen centers. Some of the smaller communities also have centers for seniors to get together to do a variety of activities. There are local swimming pools, fitness centers, public libraries, and the YWCA and YMCA. If you don't know what is available, check with your city or county services and ask.

You can also check into educational opportunities. Community colleges and universities often offer courses specifically for seniors. Public schools are often looking for volunteers to help with a variety of positions. Libraries also look for volunteers to assist in different capacities. Senior centers often host various courses or have speakers come in to teach on various topics. Maybe you have a special skill that you can teach others.

Remember: do not lose contact with your social supports. As we have already discussed, social interaction is a very important part of a healthy lifestyle. We all need to have social stimulation in our lives to survive. Research has shown this in many different studies. Gain control of your environment. Make plans and get active.

CHAPTER 5
USING LEISURE TO FIGHT DEPRESSION

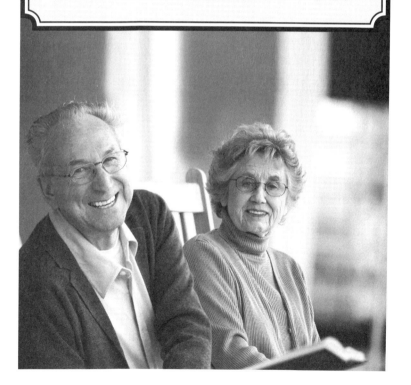

CHAPTER 5

Using Leisure to Fight Depression

D epression is more than just feeling down or sad (which we all experience from time to time in our lives). Clinical depression or major depressive disorders impact all aspects of daily life. Depression can affect everything from eating, sleeping, and working to relationships and self-esteem. People who are clinically depressed cannot simply snap out of it. Many people feel that depression is a form of mental instability. This is definitely not the case. Research has shown that medications help by treating a chemical imbalance in the brain. Depression is not a normal part of aging. It is, however, very common in the elderly. According to the WebMD website, which collaborates with the Cleveland Clinic, depression affects over six million Americans over the age of sixty-five. Only 10 percent will receive treatment because symptoms are often confused with the effects of multiple illnesses and medications. Clinical depression can be triggered by illnesses like diabetes, heart disease, stroke, cancer, Alzheimer's disease, Parkinson's disease, chronic lung disease, and arthritis. Older adults who suffer from depression are more likely to commit suicide. In fact, they account for 19 percent of all suicide deaths, according to an article written by Kevin Caruso on the website, Suicide. org.

A recent study done in Atlantic Canada found that "loneliness, finances, health, lack of transportation, and loss of family and friends are the prime causes of depression in older people living in rural areas." The project is called "Aging Well in Rural Places." Many other researchers in this field have found similar results in most of America.

Depression can be easily identified if you know what to look for. If you or someone you love is experiencing any of the following symptoms, you may want to get medical attention. Depression is a serious physical matter.

THE SIGNS AND SYMPTOMS OF DEPRESSION INCLUDE:

- Loss of interest in daily activities or activities that once brought pleasure.

- Depressed mood – feelings of sadness, helplessness, or hopelessness.

- Sleep disturbances – either sleeping too much or having problems falling asleep, waking up in the middle of the night or early morning and not being able to get back to sleep.

- Difficulty concentrating or thinking – difficulty making decisions, loss of memory.

- An increased or decrease appetite, unexplained weight loss or weight gain.

- Feelings of restlessness, agitation, or getting easily annoyed.

- Lack of energy – feeling just as tired in the morning as when going to bed the night before, feeling as if everything is in slow motion.

- Feelings of worthlessness or guilt.

- Decreased interest in sexual activities.

- Thoughts of death, dying, or suicide.

MOST OF THESE symptoms should be present for at least two weeks before being considered signs of depression. A wide variety of physical complaints can accompany depression, and those can include gastrointestinal problems, anxiety, headaches, or backaches.

Depression in the elderly often happens in conjunction with other ailments or disabilities, which can sometimes make depression difficult to diagnose. People who have experienced a stroke or heart attack have a much higher depression rate. In fact, depression is often a secondary result of the diagnosis.

Reporting symptoms of depression can help physicians treat the depression as soon as they make the diagnosis, but if those symptoms are not being reported then the chances of having depression for a long period of time increase, and recovery can take much longer. Social isolation becomes an increasing concern. Often people with these symptoms do not want to be seen in public. Social stimulation and acceptance of the disability are a good start to recovery.

There are many losses that the elderly endure. These losses may include the death of a spouse or siblings, retirement, or having to change residences. Furthermore, at this stage in life, many friends begin to pass away and the social support system that was once very plentiful starts to dwindle. Other losses include losing one's driver's license and the freedom, flexibility, and independence that a driver's license provides.

Oftentimes, caregivers are overlooked in the process of dealing with the patient. Caregivers are also at high risk of being socially isolated and suffering from depression. Someone very close to me is currently dealing with a loved one who suffers from Parkinson's disease. Although the patient is dealing with many losses that come from the disease process, the caregiver is also dealing with loss of freedom, loss of independence, decreased opportunities for social stimulation, and the loss of their loved one! It is difficult to go from the role of spouse to that of caregiver without having to deal with the loss of the relationship as it had once been. There can be anger and resentment and often no one to talk to about such feelings. I would like to take this opportunity to tell caregivers that if at all possible, I believe it would be very beneficial for you to find, or even start, a support group for caregivers. Whether it can be done through the existing support groups like the Parkinson's Society, the Alzheimer's Society, or even your local senior center, I believe it allows the opportunity to be with others that are experiencing the same things you are and may offer some very valuable tips and experiences. My heart truly aches for the caregivers. It is so important to look after yourself when you are faced with the caregiving role.

SEEKING MEDICAL ADVICE for depression is of utmost importance. Medications are useful, and the earlier the diagnosis is made, the sooner the healing process can begin. It often takes several weeks for the medications to start to work, so the sooner you can get started, the faster the relief from the symptoms.

Exercise can be very beneficial when trying to combat depression. Research has shown that exercise is often underused to treat mild to moderate depression. Exercise is effective as it helps to increase the metabolism rate as well as increase endorphins—the agents in the brain that help us "feel good." Exercise can also help with self-esteem and give us back a sense of purpose. Exercise also helps to relieve stress and anxiety and can help to improve sleep. When I deal with people who are admitted to the hospital with severe depression, I find that it often takes a couple of weeks for the medications to start working; then, I am able to get them to be more active on a social level. Sometimes it takes a lot of convincing and encouragement, but when they do start to get active, they begin to feel better and are able to begin socializing again. Persistence is the key to getting involved in life again. I know through experience that it can be extremely difficult to engage in life when all you feel like you want to do is wither up and die. I know what it feels like to not want to wake up in the morning and have to deal with another day. I also know that it takes an extreme amount of energy to get motivated to do anything. Believe me when I say that life is so worthwhile and good. Whenever a negative thought pops into your head, dismiss it and replace it with a good thought. Try this as often as you can, and think about changing your thinking pattern during the day.

Find activities that make you feel good. Start by doing something small and building up your repertoire of activities over several days. It may start with taking the dog for a walk or walking to the nearest store to buy a cup of coffee. Or it may be calling a friend whom you haven't talked to for a while. Go to the mall and window-shop for a couple of hours. Do whatever it takes to give yourself positive things to focus on throughout the day. Try not to focus on the negative thoughts that intrude on everything you do. Try using humor, whenever possible, to lighten your mood. Try to stay away from reading the newspaper as it will likely only report bad news. Instead of watching the news on TV, try watching a good sitcom, or go to the local video store and rent some good comedies. Read some feel-good books or try meditation and self-help books. There are some wonderful motivational materials out there if you are open to reading or listening to them. Remember that your ability to concentrate may be diminished, so you may need to review the material several times in order to get the best results.

> **Do whatever it takes to give yourself positive things throughout the day.**

Proper nutrition is also of utmost importance. This is especially true for those who have no appetite. Try to eat meals that are filled with nutrients rather than food that holds no nutritional value, like fast food or junk food. Tea and toast don't really provide much nourishment. Try to cook meals that will last for several days. As a very last resort, try TV dinners that can be reheated or use supplements if necessary, but your body needs to have adequate nourishment in order to function properly. Go out for meals with family members or a friend. This will provide social stimulation and an opportunity for proper nourishment.

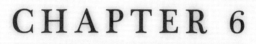

CHAPTER 6

IDENTIFYING YOUR
SUPPORT SYSTEM

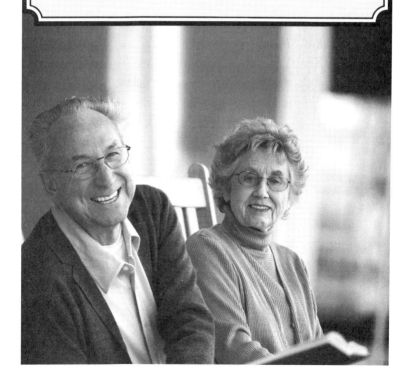

CHAPTER 6

Identifying Your Support System

Support systems are an important part of well-being. These are the people we turn to when we need understanding, encouragement, honest feedback, and assistance of any kind. It is estimated that 70 percent of the total support we receive comes from informal sources, mainly spouses and children. These represent four basic types of support: IADL (independent activities of daily living), which include shopping, personal care, transportation, and housework; emotional, which includes reassurance, comforting, confiding, and just "being there"; informational, which provides advice on seeking medical intervention, and agency referrals; and financial or housing. Support systems may include family, friends, neighbors, co-workers, or professionals. These people contribute to your life in many different ways. Reaching out for assistance can be very empowering. Reaching out can help you nourish yourself and build bridges with others. Your spouse is most likely to be your biggest support system of all. This is the one person who likely wants the very best for you in all aspects of life. When one's spouse is not well or is not functioning as well as he or she could be, it is very difficult to watch. We feel the need to do something and would probably change the world for them if we could. Our spouses are our biggest confidants, the people we have spent years with and know probably better than anyone else. Every aspect of our life involves our partner, so when there are deficits, we rely on each other to be of assistance. Participating in life together supports both parties and builds a bond that transcends other relationships; we play together and weep together. Some suggest that there is a hierarchy when older people select their social support network. They prefer to receive support from spouses first, then from children, followed by other relatives, friends, neighbors, and lastly, professional services. This has been called the hierarchical compensatory model in an article written by MJ Penning from the Centre of Aging, University of Manitoba, Winnipeg.

Another model suggests that responses requiring proximity, such as an emergency, are best handled by neighbors. Social and leisure activities are often enjoyed with friends. Supportive services that require larger investments of time and energy are done by those who have the most intimate relationships with the older person, such as children or a spouse. Once personal care needs become too overwhelming, professional services are often required. Institutionalization is the last resort. The principle of this model is that support functions are shared across a wide base of providers with each component doing what it is best suited to do.

Children are a good support system, although it may be more difficult if they do not live in close proximity. Even being in contact by phone can offer emotional and moral support. Children may arrange and pay for in-home care or move their parents to live nearer to them in order to provide the necessary care. Most adult children have a long-term commitment to their parents and search for the best alternatives that can provide the care their parents need. Some suggest that receiving too much support from children may cause distress among older people. In most Western cultures, older people prefer to be functionally separate for as long as possible before they need to rely on adult children for support. In fact, studies have shown that the elderly expect less in terms of support from their children than what the children are willing to provide. Research has suggested that well-intentioned family members who provide inappropriate amounts of assistance can actually undermine the autonomy and self-esteem of the one they are trying to care for. If the support is excessive, it can make the recipient feel guilty, incompetent, coerced, resentful, and helpless.

> Some suggest that receiving too much support from children may cause distress among older people.

Siblings are often at the same age group as the person requiring care and may or may not be able to provide the support necessary to keep living in the community. They may be able to provide emotional and social support, but may not be able to perform some of the other care needs that are required. If they are within close proximity, they are often a good resource for social stimulation and advice. It is important to note that when providing social support, one needs to be sensitive to the expectations of the older person and allow them challenges so that they can maintain skills which enable them to make a contribution to their care. This will afford a greater sense of well-being by providing a productive social role and a sense of purpose.

Friends can be a very good source of support, especially if they have been close friends for a long period of time. Because friends are often in the same age group, they also may be too frail to help with basic care needs but can serve as surrogate family members when the need arises. Close friends are often available to help share personal things, such as happy memories and tears that have been shared over the years.

Casual friendships can also be a good source of social stimulation. These friendships can afford opportunities for helping one another, such as providing transportation to appointments, social outings, shopping, attending church, banking, and other necessities. Casual friendship support can come from people whom you have met through church or other organizations such as a senior center.

Neighbors can provide assistance when emergency situations arise. Their proximity allows for a quick response to help out in times of immediate need. Neighbors can range from people you have known for a long period of time to those you wave at because you recognize them, to those you have never met. Nowadays, it seems like we hardly take the time to get to know our neighbors. We may know them to see them, but little more than that. Historically, people knew just about everyone in their neighborhood, but with the time limitations imposed on families with both the husband and wife having to work, there appears to be little time left for socializing with neighbors. Once retirement comes, it is a little easier to take the time to get to know neighbors. This can be beneficial in that you can recognize problems when they occur around you.

Your family physician can also be a wonderful source of support. Certainly, from a medical perspective, he should know you pretty well. We often go to our physician when we are very ill and in need of medical attention, but when they take the time and effort, they can get to know us on a more personal level. When they take the time, they are better able to detect ailments such as depression, anxiety, increased stress levels, and cognitive decline. If your doctor is able to discern the early symptoms of the more "difficult to assess" issues, earlier intervention can prevent further problems.

It is sometimes helpful to write down a list of your concerns before you go to see your physician as it is easy to forget all that ails you once you start talking to your doctor. Get a family member to go with you if you think you may forget some things that the doctor has said to you, or just to be sure, write them down as well. It is easy to get out of the office and remember that there was something you forgot to ask. Be prepared when you go to see your doctor. They can be real allies in getting you care. Be honest with your physicians. They are not able to help you if you do not "tell it like it is." If you are not sure about some of your symptoms, then that is a good time to have family there with you because they can fill in what we tend to forget or simply do not see.

Health care providers and home care workers who come to help perform tasks in your home can also be advocates. They are in a position to see your struggles and concerns first hand. They could be in a position to advocate for further services or to help get proper treatments. Often they are a welcome addition to the day. They provide opportunities for social stimulation in addition to the physical, emotional, and social support they provide.

You may decide you need to hire an outside agency to help with things like housekeeping, assistance with meals, or outdoor tasks like lawn and garden care and snow removal. In our community, meals-on-wheels offers services to people who have difficulty cooking for themselves or are possibly not receiving proper nourishment. Some home care services provide occupational or physical therapy in the home. These services help keep us functioning at a better level so that we are able to manage our daily activities.

OTHER SUPPORTIVE GROUPS can come through professional services. Psychologists, counselors, clergy, and other organized groups offer support in different ways. Depending on your needs, a variety of services are at your disposal. Often, counseling is a great help to people dealing with losses of many kinds, including relationships, health, and the great many other losses that we deal with as we age. You may belong to various groups, clubs, or organizations that provide support— possibly the people that you play bridge with or a coffee group, or your woodworking class. There are always people to talk to and compare notes with. These acquaintances and friends can provide comfort and a needed ear to from time to time.

They may have advice to give or just sympathize with you. Co-workers, peers, and even your boss could be good resources and sources of support. Volunteer placements offer opportunities to be with other people. This can become a place of social and emotional support and an enriching environment where your needs can be met while you are helping others. Listen to what others are saying and feeling. Maybe you are the one who can be a wonderful support for someone else. Giving support yourself is a rewarding experience.

Look around you. How many faces are familiar to you? How many people do you think would support you and your life decisions or give you good advice? How many people do you come into contact with on a daily basis? Just think of how many people are in your life. Utilizing these resources as a support system is a valuable tool in securing good relationships, counteracting social isolation, and maintaining your well-being.

Life is like a game of cards. The hand that is dealt you represents determinism; the way you play it is free will.

—Jawaharal Nehru

CHAPTER 7

GET EXCITED
ABOUT LIFE

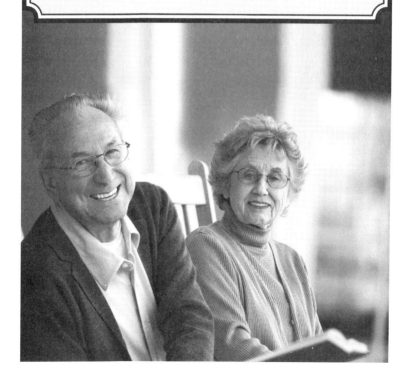

CHAPTER 7

Get Excited About Life

Nothing can stop the man with the right mental attitude from achieving his goal; nothing on earth can help the man with the wrong mental attitude.

—Thomas Jefferson

Before you go to sleep at night, think of at least one thing for which you are grateful. It doesn't matter what it is. It can be something so small that it does not seem important, just as long as you are grateful for it. As each day progresses and you continue with this practice, it will amaze you how grateful you become for so many things in your life, and your life will be more fulfilling.

The aging population continues to grow, and soon the baby boomers will be reaching retirement. Those born between 1946 and 1964 are considered baby boomers, although some historians feel that those born between 1946 and 1966 comprise the baby boom generation. Whatever years are selected, this population is growing older and will soon reach retirement age.

The implications of this are that society will soon be focused on the care of this generation and the services they need. With the increase in good medical treatment, people are living longer, and we are able to live a more fulfilling life. The medical profession is able to keep people healthy longer through new and improved medical techniques and cures. They are better able to diagnose problems, and treatment can begin earlier. There is an increased awareness of healthy lifestyle choices. We know that smoking is not healthy and that proper nutrition and exercise help us keep fit. We are also aware that good mental health is important for our well-being. There is more research being done all of the time that proves that our awareness and pursuit of healthy living improves our quality of life as we age.

I see elderly people who fashion healthy and vibrant lifestyles, and those who fashion detrimental lifestyles, and the quality of life and physical health in both are evident. Some people who are in their eighties look like they are in their seventies, and some who are sixty look like they are in their eighties or nineties. Some people have lived very hard lives, which is evident in their physical appearance. We now experience much easier living conditions than those of our grandparents and even those of our parents. We have not had to endure the physical hardships that they did when they were growing up. We live in a time when most things come fairly easily. The government assists those who are having difficulties, but for the most part there is ample food and shelter for us. Technology has provided us with many things that make our lives easier. Washing machines were a luxury for my parents' generation. My mother was very happy to have a wringer washer when I was a kid. We now have computers, automobiles, jet airplanes, and many other conveniences. Living and leisure conditions have improved significantly over the past century, and it is difficult to envision what the next century will bring.

Have you ever heard the expression "age is just a state of mind"? Well, it is true! You are as old as you feel! Some days, when I feel run down and tired, I feel much older than I actually am, but my spirit always feels young and vibrant. I love life and all that it offers, even the bad. Without the bad things that happen to us, how would we know when we are experiencing the good things? I believe that if we can focus on the good and be grateful for what we have, we can begin to see things in a more positive light. When we focus on the bad events, we draw more bad to ourselves. Think about it—when you start off the day on a bad note, it seems the rest of the day is bad. If we overcome that one bad event, we can change the way the rest of the day goes for us.

We need to look after our mind, body, and spirit and feed them daily so that we can live life to the fullest. I was sent the following story on the Internet, and I think it is very fitting.

I got to thinking one day about all those women on the Titanic who passed up dessert at dinner that fateful night in an effort to cut back. From then on, I've tried to be a little more flexible. How many women out there will eat at home because their husband didn't suggest going out to dinner until after something had been thawed? Does the word "refrigeration" mean nothing to you? How often have your kids dropped in to talk and sat in silence while you watched "Jeopardy!" on television? I cannot count the times I called my sister and said, "How about going to lunch in a half hour?" She would stammer, "I can't. I have clothes on the line. My hair is dirty. I wish I had known yesterday. I had a late breakfast. It looks like rain," and my personal favorite, "It's Monday." She died a few years ago and we never did have lunch together.

Because we cram so much into our lives, we tend to schedule our headaches. We live on a sparse diet of promises we make to ourselves when all the conditions are perfect! We'll go back and visit the grandparents when we get little Johnny toilet-trained,

> We live on a sparse diet of promises we make to ourselves when all the conditions are perfect!

or we'll entertain when we replace the living room carpet, or maybe we'll go on a second honeymoon when we get two more kids out of college. Life has a way of accelerating as we get older. The days get shorter, and the list of promises to ourselves gets longer. One morning, we wake and all we have to show for our lives is a litany of "I'm going to ... I plan on ... and, someday, when things settle down a bit."

When anyone calls my "seize the moment" friend, she is open to adventure and available for trips. She keeps an open mind to new ideas. Her enthusiasm for life is contagious. You talk with her for five minutes and you're ready to trade your bad feet for a pair of rollerblades and skip an elevator for a bungee cord.

My lips have not touched ice cream in ten years. I love ice cream. It's just that I might as well apply it directly to my stomach with a spatula and eliminate the digestive process. The other day, I stopped the car and bought a triple-decker. If my car had hit an iceberg on the way home, I would have died happy.

Now, go on and have a nice day. Do something you want to, not something on your "should do" list. If you were going to die soon and had only one phone call you could make, who would you call and what would you say? And why are you waiting?

Have you ever watched kids playing on a merry-go-round or listened to the rain lapping on the ground? Ever followed a butterfly's erratic flight or gazed at the sun into the fading night? Do you run through each day on the fly? When you ask, "How are you?" do you hear the reply? When the day is done, do you lie in your bed with the next hundred chores running through your head? Ever told your child, "We'll do it tomorrow," and in your haste not seen his or her sorrow? Ever lost touch, or let a good friendship die? Ever just call to say, "Hi?"

When you worry and hurry though your day, it is like an unopened gift that has been thrown away. Life is not a race, so take is slower and hear the music before the song is over. Life may not be the party we hoped for, but while we are here, we might as well dance!

GET EXCITED ABOUT LIFE

—**Author Unknown**

LIFE IS ABOUT being and living. It's your attitude that can make the biggest difference. If you believe that the world is an evil place, guess what? For you, the world will become an evil place. On the other hand, if you see that the world provides opportunities for learning and growing and that, for the most part, other people are good, then you will tend to be a happier individual. Sometimes it can be a struggle to see things in your life as being good, but we all learn through our experiences.

We learn wisdom from failure much more than success. We often discover what we will do, by finding out what we will not do.

—**Samuel Smiles**

LIFE IS WHAT you make of it. It is the choices you make and what you wish to learn in your time on this Earth. We have been given the right to make many choices in our lives, and those choices can bring us great wealth and happiness. You can attract positive events and positive people into your life with your positive energy. People want to be around people who are happy and live life with energy and verve. Do you want to hang around someone who is negative all the time and who does nothing but complain about ailments and unpleasant things in his or her life? I know that I don't! I get more positive energy from happy and positive people.

I worked with a lady who had the most arthritic and deformed fingers I had ever seen. You would think that she would complain about the pain and the inability to perform tasks, but she would spend hours in her room doing fine needle work! She loved being with people and socializing and doing crafts. She needed some help with certain activities, but she was more than willing to try anything. She was an inspiration to me! There are others, however, who feel that their arthritic fingers should allow them to refuse to participate in activities. It has been proven that moving your arthritic fingers and hands can actually be beneficial and help to decrease the pain. Attitude can really make the difference as to how you view your world.

If you don't have access to the things that you feel are important to your well-being, let your needs be known. Get involved in groups and clubs that can make a difference! Find out what other people feel are important issues as well. There are many opportunities to lobby for the activities that you feel are needed in your community. If nobody says anything, then nothing will get done. Let your voice be heard and make a difference in your community.

WRITE TO YOUR local MLA or other government agencies. They are often the ones who make the decisions regarding funding. The squeaky wheel gets the grease, and the more noise you make, the better your chances of getting what you want. Be persistent! Get others on your side, and work together as a team. It will give you a sense of purpose and provide the opportunity to do something of value for your community. How exciting is that?

Talk to family and friends. Make a plan, and get out there and do it. Life has so much to offer, but you need to take the opportunities that are given to you. You are the master of your own well-being. No one can do it for you. Sometimes you need to be a little bit creative, but if you really set your mind to doing something, I have no doubt in my mind that you can. If you had asked me five years ago if I would ever write a book, I would have said that was not very likely. Well, here I am sharing my knowledge and experiences with you. If I can do this, then you can do anything you chose to do! Learning new skills and expanding your knowledge is never out of reach. Some say that you can't teach an old dog new tricks, but I beg to differ. I hear seniors all the time who say that they have learned something new that day, whether it was a new craft, idea, or activity. There is no end to the possibilities of what can be learned.

There are adaptations and modifications that can be done to recreational activities to make them accessible if you need special accommodations. I have seen bowling alleys that provide ramps for wheelchair bowling, large numbers on playing cards so they are easier to read, books on tape for those who can't read, and plastic canvas sewing for those who have trouble with small needles and thread. Many communities offer transportation services that allow for wheelchairs or walkers and provide better access to their facilities. Every time you think of something you can't do, try to think instead, "How can I do this?" Stedman Graham said, "People who consider themselves victims of their circumstances will always remain victims unless they develop a greater vision for their lives."

TAKE A COURSE at your local college or university. What have you always wanted to know more about? It could be a recreational or leisure activity, or it could be a course in public speaking or technical writing. Maybe you would like to earn a diploma or degree. You will likely not use this degree to find yourself a job, but it is an accomplishment! What a feeling to accomplish something that you have set your heart and mind on doing.

Teaching others can also provide a sense of accomplishment. Maybe you could help out at a local school. You could read to young kids and talk to them about your life experiences.

What have you accomplished in your life? Would others benefit from your experiences? What can you teach children or young adults? If you feel that what you have learned or experienced in your life can be beneficial, offer your services.

What can you learn from your peers? Do you share the same experiences that you can talk about, or do you have varying experiences that are interesting to talk about with others? What can you teach your peers about life, about opportunities, about activity choices? Are you a caregiver who can give advice to other caregivers? Could you start a support group for others in the same circumstances that you are in?

There are many ways to help others and teach each other. Look for those opportunities. Hospitals and nursing homes are always looking for volunteers to help out in many areas. There is a woman who comes to our unit every Monday just to visit. She goes from room to room to see if anyone would like to visit for a while. She feels that what she has to offer is a valuable service to the patients that she sees. We have volunteers who bring their dogs in to visit, volunteers who play music or sing, and volunteers who help with recreational activities or church services. Maybe you have a special skill that you can teach to others. You have so much to offer to others. You just need to tap into your knowledge base and be willing to share it.

Spending time with family is such a great way to experience life. Sharing time with your own children or grandchildren can be such a rewarding experience. I love spending time with my grandchildren. It is a chance to do things with them that I may not have been able to afford to do when my own children were younger. So, if you have grandchildren, take them to a park or zoo, spoil them rotten, or just sit and play with them. I remember when I was a teenager, I would occasionally go to visit my grandmother by myself. She would tell me stories of her youth, and I found it interesting to know that she had some of the same experiences that I had. She talked about being late for school because she and her friends were busy playing by the river and other antics from her childhood.

It helps to have someone to listen to, and grandparents make a pretty good sounding board. The advice that young teens or children seek may not be from a parent, but from someone who is nonjudgmental as they are more distant from the issues and problems. Most kids look up to seniors as a source of guidance and unconditional love. They really enjoy it if you can take the time to attend activities and events that they are involved in. This past Christmas, I attended my oldest grandson's first Christmas concert. It brought back memories of my own children and their concerts, but it also felt good to see so many very young faces trying their very best to perform for their families. What a joy and blessing grandchildren can be to us.

You need to find out what gives you life and vitality. What do you enjoy doing? Do you like being active, or do you prefer being more passive? Do you like being socially active? Do you enjoy crafts, woodworking, playing pool, or perhaps swimming?

Identifying what you enjoy doing is a good start to finding out what gives you the motivation to get out of bed and participate in life.

You should also ask yourself what you do to feel energized and vital. How can you incorporate those things into your life now? What did you do when you were a child that gave you that feeling? What about when you were in your twenties, thirties, or forties? Is there a fear in your life that you want to conquer? I try every morning to wake up and imagine that my day is filled with all things that are positive and to look forward to that day. I imagine the very best outcome and proceed to make my day progress as well as I had imagined or better.

Think about the last time you felt like shouting, "YAHOO!" and what you were doing at the time. I call this the yahoo factor. What gives you that yahoo factor? When you accomplish a difficult task, do you feel that yahoo factor? When you go to the gym or for a walk or win a game of tennis, do you feel the yahoo factor? I get the yahoo factor from achieving a goal that I have set for myself. I get the yahoo factor when I watch my husband race his sprint car and finish in the top places. I get it when I climb to the top of a hiking trail. There are many ways and opportunities to find your yahoo factor. Doesn't it feel good? Don't you want to feel that more often in your life? Go for it! Live your life to the fullest, and experience the fulfillment and well-being that you are entitled to.

You can learn more about a man in an hour of play than in a lifetime of conversation.

—Plato

CHAPTER 8

MOTIVATE
YOURSELF

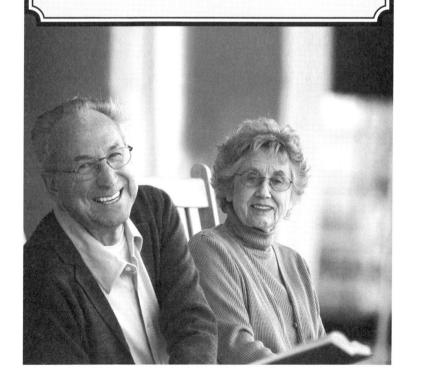

CHAPTER 8

Motivate Yourself

People become really quite remarkable when they start thinking that they can do things. When they believe in themselves, they have the first secret of success.

- Norman Vincent Peale

The things that motivate us often come from the things that we need in life. The needs of seniors have been identified as follows: the need for acknowledgement, shelter, nourishment, income, health, safety, socialization, respect, education, meaningful activity/recreation, and independence.

In 1943, Abraham Maslow proposed a "Theory of Human Motivation," which is often shown as a pyramid consisting of five levels. His theory suggests a progression of needs that can only proceed to the next level when the first has been accomplished, and as one moves up through the stages, the needs in the lower levels are no longer a priority.

The first level of the pyramid consists of the physiological needs. These include the need for oxygen, food, water, and a stable body temperature. These are the strongest needs, and if these are not met, it will not be possible to progress to the next level.

The second level consists of safety needs. When all the physiological needs are met and are no longer at the forefront of our thoughts and behaviors, the need for security becomes a priority. These needs include security, order, law, stability, and protection from the elements. We have little awareness of our need for safety except in times of emergency.

When these needs are met, we can then move on to the next phase in the process. The third level is comprised of the need for love, affection, and belonging. This involves both giving and receiving love and affection in many contexts, including work groups, family, friendships, and intimate sexual relationships. Love and affection can come from a large social group or from small social connections. There is a need to love and to be loved by others. When these needs are not met, people are more susceptible to social anxiety, loneliness, and depression.

Maslow also identifies the need for esteem. This involves the need for self-esteem and for the esteem that one person gets from another. These allow one to feel confident and valuable as a person. All humans have a need to have self-respect and feel respect for others. People need to have a chance to contribute, to gain recognition, and to take part in activities that provide opportunities to feel accepted and valued. However, it is important to recognize that people must first accept themselves internally.

The last step in the motivational pyramid is the need for self-actualization. Only when all other needs have been satisfied can people achieve what they were "born to do." This is when people can realize their potential, achieve self-fulfillment, and seek personal growth and experiences. Such people can now become mature human beings and fulfill their desires to realize all of their potential for being effective and creative. Maslow identifies self-actualized people in the following ways: they embrace the facts and realities of the world; they are spontaneous, creative, and interested in solving problems; they feel close to other people and appreciate life; they have a system of morality that is internalized; and they are able to view all things objectively.

These are the basic behaviors that Maslow believes motivate us. You will not be able to move upwards until you are successful in meeting the needs of the previous step, and depending on which step of the process you are in, this will have different implications. It should be noted that we can, and often do, fluctuate between the steps depending on circumstances in our lives.

One of the goals of achievement is being successful. Success is composed of three areas—skill, knowledge, and attitude. Skill is about 5 percent of what it takes to achieve our goals. About 10 percent comes from knowledge and effort, and the remaining 85 percent boils down to attitude. Hard to believe, isn't it, that such a huge percentage of how we can achieve success is based on attitude? Success is the progressive realization of a worthy goal. Our attitude and value system can be the major stumbling block or greatest catalyst to success.

There are people out there with little formal education who have gone on to achieve success in their lives by owning companies or becoming brilliant musicians. That is because they are motivated to achieve, and no one is going to tell them they can't succeed. They have set their goals and will strive to reach these goals. The skills that they have are limited, but their hearts are filled with drive and determination, and that will often overcome lack of skill. We are human beings that can learn and make choices based on our perceptions of our own needs.

Knowledge is a tool for getting us where we want to go. Our knowledge about certain things can lead us in a certain direction and help us to make the decisions that are based on that particular knowledge.

> **Knowledge is a tool for getting us where we want to go.**

At the age of twenty-four, I spent many hours researching my career alternatives. I made the decision to become a recreation therapist. I knew that I loved working with seniors and wanted to make a career out of it. The knowledge I gained through researching alternatives helped me to make the choice to participate in an educational experience that changed my life. When I made this decision to go back to school, I had three children who were three, four, and five years old. Nevertheless, I made up my mind that I was going to graduate with honors. This was very difficult at times. I found myself staying up until midnight doing papers and getting up at five in the morning to study for exams because those were the quietest times. My attitude towards my goal helped me to achieve what I had set out to do. I believed in myself and my intellect to get the job done.

It is kind of like trying to quit smoking. I know there are many people out there who have tried many times and keep failing despite all of the drugs and programs designed to help people quit. I feel a mental attitude is the most powerful tool in trying to quit smoking. I tried many times to quit; however, I really enjoyed smoking. It wasn't until I set a date and really decided that I was going to quit for good that I managed to quit. It has been nearly six years, and I have never had another cigarette. Call it willpower, determination, or whatever name you chose to give it. It is your attitude towards your goals that will make a difference in your life.

It is important to realize that our attitudes and values determine how much we actually want to achieve success. Sometimes our attitudes can be a huge barrier to achieving what we are striving for. If you have a negative attitude, well, chances are that you will not achieve success because you have already told yourself that it is unattainable. Your attitude will have a significant impact on how you can overcome any barriers to your success. Face it, there will always be wrenches thrown into your best-laid plans, but how you handle those difficulties and barriers will determine whether or not you achieve your goals. Zig Zigler said it well when he said, "The difference between a big shot and a little shot is that a big shot's just a little shot that kept on shooting."

A patient that I worked with came up to talk to me during one of our music programs and said, "Have you noticed that lots of the other people around here have such an angry look on their faces when they come out of their rooms?" I told her that I really hadn't noticed, but as I started to look around, she was right. She proceeded to spend the next hour listening to the music, swaying her hips, tapping her toes and singing to the music. She was upbeat, pleasant, and such a joy to be around. She was ninety-four years old and had the spirit of someone so much younger. I decided that I want to be like her when I am ninety-four years old. I want to surround myself with positive people who are happy, walk with smiles on their faces, and dance to music.

As you think, so shall you be! Think about it. Do you think you are a vibrant, successful person that is filled with life and passion, or do you believe that you are a loser and not worthy of anything in your life? You need to change the way you think about yourself! The more positive your attitude, the more positive events and people you will draw into your life. The same principal applies to a negative attitude. This is called the Law of Attraction. Basically, positive attracts positive and negative attracts negative. Do you like being around negative people? I certainly don't. I would much prefer to be in an environment where I can feel good and secure and happy in what life has to offer. If everyone around you is negative and unhappy and constantly complaining, well, after a while it gets very monotonous, and you do not want to be in the presence of these people for very long. If you think positive thoughts, you will attract positive things. Additionally, when confronted with negativity, you will be much better served to remove yourself from that situation, if possible, and look for positive people to be around.

Have you ever noticed that if you are sitting with a small group of people and someone starts talking about negative events in his or her life, others tend to follow in that same train of thought, and soon everyone in that group feels downtrodden and negative? Every bad event in our lives has something good in it, but sometimes it can be difficult to find. Maybe it is a lesson learned or maybe an avenue to something even better. Dave Garner said that success is getting what you want, and happiness is wanting what you get.

SETTING GOALS IS a good way to motivate ourselves to achieve success. It can be a very large goal, but break it down into bite-sized pieces. When you take the time to write your goals down, you are making a mental commitment to completing them. It means that you are actually taking the time to commit your thoughts and desires to paper, making them more meaningful and powerful. It is difficult to ignore your goals when you face them every day, and that's exactly where you need to put them—in a prominent place where you have visual contact with them frequently. It is far easier to think about your dreams and goals, but it becomes significant when you write them down!

You need to decide what constitutes success in your life. No one else can do it for you—just like no one can make you quit smoking or make you run a marathon. If you have the desire and drive to do something, then it will get done. Simple, isn't it? Try it and see. You may be amazed at the results!

Making decisions and choices can be difficult at times. Start by investigating your options and what you may need to make happen in order to achieve the results that you are looking for. Research all the avenues that are available to you. Start by looking at your past and what was meaningful to you then. Then, look at your present and the things that meet your needs. Then determine what you may want to try to achieve in the future.

You also need to determine what constitutes success in your life. Does success mean increased health and wellness, meaningful relationships, increased social opportunities, or improving money management skills? You must feel that what you are doing in your life fits into your definition of success. I may determine that I will be successful when I have lost thirty pounds, but that most likely is not the same thing to which you aspire. At different times in our lives, our needs are different. When we observe Maslow's hierarchy of needs, it shows how we are motivated by our needs and that we can move between the different levels depending on circumstances in our life.

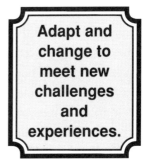

Adapt and change to meet new challenges and experiences.

Andrew Carnegie said, "People who are unable to motivate themselves must be content with mediocrity, no matter how impressive their other talents." In other words, if you are content with what you currently have, you will never aspire to achieve better things in your life, even if you are the most brilliant person on this earth. Without motivation and the drive to succeed, your talents will be wasted.

Adapt and change to meet new challenges and experiences. We tend to get into a rut from time to time, but I believe that every once in a while, we just need to shake things up. Be creative in how you approach life. Look at the things that you are doing, and think about how you could change them, improve on them, and adapt them if necessary. Sometimes when we look at some of the activities that we used to participate in, we may find that they may need to be adapted or changed in order to meet our needs. Look at the people who participate in the Paralympics. They include people with amputations, cerebral palsy, vision impairments, intellectual disabilities, and people in wheelchairs. What commitment and motivation each of those athletes has, especially when faced with disability! Their vision and dedication is admirable, and needs to be applauded.

Life is what you make of it. No one can motivate you except yourself. It is an internal process that you need to develop. It comes from the needs and wants in your life and the desire to make changes. When you take the time to identify your needs and wants, it will allow you to be more accurate in developing your goals. When you take time and work through the process of goal setting, your ability to motivate yourself is so much easier. You are taking the time and dedicating yourself to the process, and you will be more likely to follow through and make good on the goals you have set for yourself.

Keeping a daily log or diary will help you to notice your improvements and how you are feeling. You will be able to see your development as a process, and even though there may be only tiny steps of improvement, you will be able to identify them.

It can also help you to write down your frustrations and how you overcame some of those things in your life that tend to pull you down. Try to put a positive spin on things that seem bad. If you look hard enough, you will always find some good in things that may not seem or feel very good. The more you can focus on the good things, the easier it will be to have a positive outlook on life.

Also, share your experiences with others. We can all learn from each other, whether it be how best to do something or what is best to avoid. Vicarious learning can be very beneficial. Some of us tend to learn things the hard way, but sometimes that can be avoided if we listen to and take to heart what others have learned. That's not to say that you should never try a new experience, but maybe you could learn how to do it differently from someone else and make it a positive experience. Don't forget: We are all individuals with different sets of experience and learning styles. Some of us like to be extravagant in our learning experiences. When I think about the ninety-year-old man who wants to learn how to sky dive, or the eighty-year-old lady who bungee jumps or goes on a hot air balloon ride, it brings a huge smile to my face. Not every one of us is cut out for that.

The question for each man to settle is not what he would do if he had means, time, influence and educational advantages; the question is what he will do with the things he has. The moment a young man ceases to dream or to bemoan his lack of opportunities and resolutely looks his conditions in the face, and resolves to change them, he lays the corner-stone of a solid and honourable success.

—Hamilton Wright Mabie

LEARNING WHAT MAKES you tick or experience joy can be a fulfilling undertaking. Do you like to take risks, or do you prefer the more sedentary activities? We are all luminous beings living in human form. Our spirit is so big and bright, and we have the ability to attract all that is good into our lives. Look around you and see how many people live in this world. Look at the ones who seem healthiest and happiest. What are they doing differently from you?

People who are happiest and healthiest know where they are going in their lives and have positive attitudes. They know what brings them joy, and they follow their joy, and happiness flows through them. These are the kinds of people who attract people and events to them through the power of attraction. We all have that ability, if we choose to use it. There are so many books and tapes on motivation and how to find yourself. It could be well worth your while to look into some of these books that can help develop that wonderful power of being positive.

Being productive also helps us feel positive. We can learn to be productive in so many ways. We can help ourselves by being involved in different organizations and groups. We can help others, which in turn benefits us by boosting our self-esteem as we contribute to the well-being of others. We have so much to offer to others. Winston Churchill put it this way: "We make a living by what we get, but we make a life by what we give."

We are all social beings and need to love and to be loved. We are not all social butterflies, but we do need some social contact. Prisoners are given solitary confinement as a punishment for bad behavior. Some people choose solitary confinement, but in the end it too is only a punishment. Explore your social contacts and maintain them if at all possible. It can actually help to provide you with a longer and more fulfilling life!

It comes down to the simple saying. If you think you can, you may be right. If you think you can't, you are almost certainly right. Put another way, success comes in cans!

—John Stevens

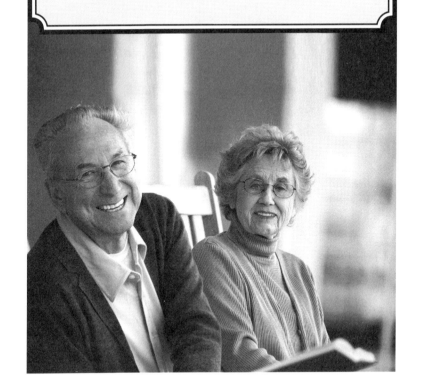

CHAPTER 9

MAKING A PLAN

CHAPTER 9

Making a Plan

Well, now comes the part where we get down to setting our goals. The first step we need to take is to identify how much free time we have in the day. What I want you to do is look at a typical day and break it down into half-hour intervals. There is a worksheet provided, so get a pen, and let's get to work.

Fill in the spaces where you have time that is dedicated to some activity, whether it is getting ready for the day, preparing a meal, watching TV programs, or even completing household tasks.

MAKING A PLAN

WORKSHEET

6:00 a.m. _____

6:30 a.m. _____

7:00 a.m. _____

7:30 a.m _____

8:00 a.m. _____

8:30 a.m. _____

9:00 a.m. _____

9:30 a.m _____

10:00 a.m. _____

10:30 a.m. _____

11:00 a.m. _____

11:30 a.m. _____

12:00 p.m. _____

1:00 p.m. _____

1:30 p.m. _____

2:00 p.m. _____

2:30 p.m. _____

3:00 p.m. _____

3:30 p.m. _____

4:00 p.m. _____

4:30 p.m. _____

5:00 p.m. _____

5:30 p.m. _____

6:00 p.m. _____

6:30 p.m. _____

7:00 p.m. _____

7:30 p.m. _____

8:00 p.m. _____

8:30 p.m. _____

9:00 p.m. _____

9:30 p.m. _____

10:00 p.m. _____

10:30 p.m. _____

11:00 p.m. _____

11:30 p.m. _____

12:00 p.m. _____

How much free time do I have?

NOW TAKE A look at the gaps in your day. What changes would you like to make in how you are spending your day?

_____

_____

_____

IS THERE ANYTHING you can do to change how you are spending your time?

_____

_____

OUR NEXT STEP is to identify our needs. Rate your needs from one to five, with one being the highest.

WHAT ARE MY NEEDS?

_____ To do something meaningful

_____ To have a feeling of belonging

_____ To meet new people

_____ To keep busy

_____ To be entertained

_____ To gain the respect of others

_____ To be successful

_____ To use my imagination

_____ To learn something new

_____ To help others

_____ To be part of a group

_____ To relax and just take it easy

_____ To be challenged

_____ To relieve stress and tension

_____ To laugh and enjoy life

_____ To be able to choose independently what I want to do

_____ To improve my fitness level

MAKING A PLAN

_____ To stimulate my mental abilities

_____ To organize myself to get motivated

_____ To be available to help family and friends

_____ To prevent loneliness

_____ To feel valued

_____ To feel good about myself

_____ To try something new and different

_____ To explore new opportunities

_____ To be productive

_____ To teach others

_____ To increase my self-esteem

_____ To be creative

_____ To be active

_____ To be a leader

_____ To feel confident

_____ To be alone

_____ To take risks

_____ To feel secure

_____ To be able to express my spirituality

_____ Other?

Specify _____

_____

_____

NOW THAT YOU have rated your needs, let's put them into perspective. Take your top five needs and write them down. On the other side of the page, identify what activities you feel would fill those needs and would be enjoyable to you. Keep in mind whether you prefer large group activities, active or passive participation. Do you want to increase your productivity or increase time for relaxation? Do you want to increase your fitness levels or cognitive abilities?

Lifestyle Needs	Activity Preferences
1. _____	1. _____
_____	2. _____
_____	3. _____
_____	
2. _____	1. _____
_____	2. _____
_____	3. _____
3. _____	1. _____
_____	2. _____

	3. _____
4. _____	1. _____
_____	2. _____
_____	3. _____
5. _____	1. _____
_____	2. _____
_____	3. _____

NOW YOU MAY look at your list and come up with a million excuses as to why you can't do these things. Let's look at some of the most common barriers to enjoying leisure experiences.

Physical limitations can be very difficult to overcome. The type of disability you have influences the types of activities you can do. If this is the case for you, you may need to be a little more creative and investigate more options. Rest assured, many of these barriers can be overcome through modifications and adaptations to the activity itself.

Lack of motivation can be a significant deterrent to contributing to your own well-being. It is an intrinsic barrier that can be very difficult to deal with. Having others around who can give you a little push every once in a while can be helpful. Remember, your attitude and how you view life can make a big difference in how you manage your goals and objectives.

Attitude: The more I live the more I understand that life in not a 50/50 proposition but rather LIFE is 10% what happens to me and 90% how I react to it.

— Anonymous

NOT HAVING ENOUGH free time is another barrier people often identify. Most seniors do not have this problem, especially when they really identify what time they have available to them. Some will say that by the time they get up, get dressed, cook, and clean the house, there is no free time left. The exercise on discovering how much free time you have can be a real eye-opener to just how much time is available to you.

Transportation can be a real issue for seniors, especially if they are no longer able to drive due to a disability or age. Some women never learned how to drive, and when their spouses die, they feel stranded. Check out your options in your community. Some people have access to wheelchair or handicapped transportation services. Others use public transportation. Some senior centers have transportation available to members for a nominal fee while others rely on family and friends.

Some people are just not aware of services that are available to them. Again, you need to investigate the options and availability of services and opportunities in your area.

IDENTIFYING BARRIERS TO YOUR ENJOYMENT

AS YOU GO through the checklist, check all the barriers that apply to you.

_____ I often don't feel like doing anything

_____ I have too many family obligations

_____ I don't think leisure is important

_____ I am not sure what is meaningful for me

_____ I am under too much stress

_____ I do not have enough money to do what I want to do

_____ I have too many physical limitations

_____ I don't have any creative or artistic skills

_____ I am embarrassed when it comes to learning new skills

_____ I have way too much work to do around the house

_____ I don't know what is available

_____ I tend to procrastinate

_____ There is no one to go with

_____ I don't like unfamiliar situations

_____ I do not get enough support from my family

_____ I don't like to make decisions about
participating in activities

_____ I have difficulties following through

_____ I enjoy activities that are not available
in my community

_____ I do not have available transportation

_____ I do not have the financial means

_____ I do not feel motivated to do anything

_____ My physical limitations prevent me
from getting involved

_____ Any other barriers that you can think of?

Identify _____

_____

_____

_____

MAKING A PLAN

NOW THAT YOU have identified your barriers, list the top five. Beside each barrier, try to list three ways you can overcome that barrier.

1. _____	1. _____
_____	2. _____
_____	3. _____
2. _____	1. _____
_____	2. _____
_____	3. _____
3. _____	1. _____
_____	2. _____
_____	3. _____
4. _____	1. _____
_____	2. _____
_____	3. _____
5. _____	1. _____
_____	2. _____
_____	3. _____

Let's take this next area just to learn a little bit about ourselves.

What are your three favorite activities?

1 _____

2. _____

3. _____

What do you enjoy most about these activities?

_____

_____

_____

What are your three least favorite activities?

1. _____

2. _____

3. _____

What do you dislike the most about doing these activities?

_____

_____

_____

How would you like to spend a Saturday afternoon?

_____

_____

_____

If you suddenly inherited a lot of money, what would you do with it?

_____

_____

_____

What are some of the activities that you enjoyed doing when you were younger?

_____

_____

_____

What activity did you do most recently that you enjoyed the most?

_____

_____

MAKING A PLAN

Finish the following sentences:

1. When I am on vacation, I like to _____

_____

2. If I had $50 to spend, I would _____

_____

3. The happiest day of my life was _____

_____

4. My favorite vacation place is _____

_____

5. When I am at home alone, I _____

_____

6. I am sad when _____

_____

7. I am very good at _____

_____

8. On rainy days I like to_____

_____

9. My favorite activity is_____

_____

10. I spend most of my time doing _____

_____

11. At night I like to_____

_____

12. On weekends I spend my time doing _____

_____

13. When I go to parties, I always _____

_____

14. I like watching movies that are _____

_____

15. I like to go out for dinner to _____

_____

16. My favorite TV shows are _____

_____

17. When it snows outside I like to _____

_____

18. When I need exercise, I _____

_____

19. Every summer I _____

_____

20. I like to read these kinds of books: _____

_____

21. I enjoy attending parties that are _____

_____

22. I enjoy being with friends when _____

_____

23. When I am feeling sad, I like to _____

_____

24. I enjoy this kind of music: _____

_____

25. When I go shopping, I like to_____

_____

THIS ACTIVITY HELPS reveal and explore attitudes, beliefs, actions, interests, convictions, aspirations, likes, and dislikes. The result of doing this activity is a new awareness of our values and motivators.

How can this be incorporated into your life now? Can you take any of these activities that you have identified here and participate in them now? Can you identify why you do some of the activities that you do?

What are the things that you enjoy doing?

1. _____

2. _____

3. _____

4. _____

5. _____

Identify family or friends that you can call or visit when you are lonely or bored.

1. _____

2. _____

3. _____

4. _____

5. _____

Identify religious organizations and/or community groups that may be available to offer you support when you need it.

1. _____

2. _____

3. _____

4. _____

5. _____

MAKING A PLAN

Identify the places that you like to go.

1. _____

2. _____

3. _____

4. _____

5. _____

YOU HAVE NOW explored a lot of different things through this process. Let's take the final step and set some goals. Goal setting is not simply writing an idea on paper.

Goals should be straightforward and state what you want to happen. They need to be specific and define what we are going to do. First, make sure that your goals are something that you really want and not just something that sounds good. We all tend to talk about what we want to do or are going to do, but it takes more commitment to write it down. This process can also make us think a little more clearly about what we really want to accomplish.

Always write your goals positively. Always write about what you want rather than what you do not want. For example:

POSITIVE:

I WILL BE involved in three different activities per week to get me out of the house and increase my social stimulation.

NEGATIVE:

I DO NOT want to be stuck in the house any more, so I will try to get out more often.

The more often we can think positively, the more positive things we attract into our lives.

Be specific in your goals. As seen by the above statement, you need to be very detailed in your goal setting. That applies to any goals that you set in your life. The more information you put into your goal, the clearer the final outcome will be.

Make sure that your goal is high enough! Don't be content with the small stuff. Bob Proctor said that if your goal is easily attainable, it is not big enough. Think big, and believe that you will achieve what you desire in your life.

Then write it down! This will help to create the map that will lead to your success. Put your written goals in a space that you will see every day. Use them as a reminder of what you want to achieve. Visualize the completed goal. This will help you get your subconscious working together with your conscious mind to help you meet your goals. Do not allow negative self-talk to get you down. Focus on how your goal will improve your life and well-being.

When you set goals that improve your quality of life, it does not matter how long the process takes as long as you continue to take steps that will take you to your final goal. The more steps you make, the happier you will be and the more fulfilling the process of achieving your goals will become.

Obstacles are what we see only when we lose sight of our goals.

— **Author Unknown**

Your action plan, or objectives, are simply the steps you are going to take to reach your goal.

EXAMPLE:

GOAL:

I am going to attend a square dancing class to help me improve my physical fitness and put me in a situation where I can socialize with others.

ACTION STEPS:

1. I will investigate the possible places I can take the class. These include the senior center, the local community college, and the local university.

2. I will enroll in the class of my choice, and one that is convenient for me.

3. I will find ways to get to the class, whether I drive, take a taxi, or ride with someone else.

4. I will be faithful in attending the class.

5. I will be open to socializing with others in the class.

SO NOW IT is your turn. What do you want to accomplish and improve in your life? Start with three goals then once they have been attained, set three more goals, then three more goals. Never quit setting goals for yourself and you will be amazed and pleasantly surprised at what you can accomplish!

SETTING YOUR GOALS

Goal #1. _____

_____

_____

_____

Action steps (how you will achieve your goal)

1. _____

2. _____

MAKING A PLAN

3. _____

4. _____

5. _____

Goal #2. _____

_____

_____

_____

Action steps

1. _____

2. _____

3. _____

4. _____

5. _____

Goal #3. _____

_____

_____

_____

Action steps

1. _____

2. _____

3. _____

4. _____

5. _____

YOU MAY FIND it helpful to highlight or cross out the action steps after you have taken them. This will show you that you are indeed on your way to achieving your goal.

Your positive thinking and willingness to make a change in your life is the first step to achieving wellness and an improved quality of life. You are the only one who can change how you think and how you are. There is not one other person in the universe who can get into your mind or soul and change you. Your attitude and how you relate to the world make you who you are. What you attract into your being and into your world is what determines how you live. Think positive thoughts, take the steps required to reach your goals, and you will achieve success. You have the power to reach out and feel good about who you are. You have the power to find enrichment and fulfillment in your life.

When you reach your goals, it is like standing on the highest mountain and looking around, knowing that you accomplished something great in your life! You can feel good about who you are, and when you can feel good about yourself, it is easy to feel good about those around you too. Others will notice an improvement in you, and you will be able to give so much more of yourself, both to yourself and others.

You can't hit a home run unless you step up to the plate. You can't catch fish unless you put your line in the water. You can't reach your goals if you don't try.

— **Kathy Seligman**

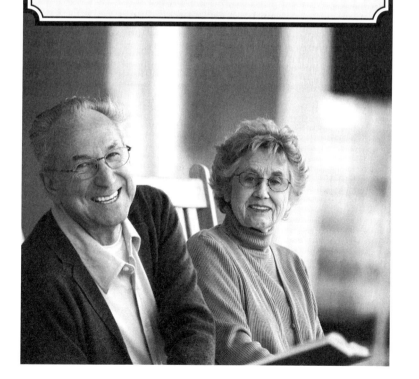

CHAPTER 10

RECOMMENDED RESOURCES

CHAPTER 10

Recommended Resources

The resources listed in this chapter are only a very small sample of what is available. They have been broken down into U.S. resources, Canadian resources, and general resources. They are listed first, and in case you require further information, it is included further in the chapter. Many Canadian organizations are provincial and therefore have not been mentioned here. For example, Meals on Wheels operates in Canada as well as the United States, but in Canada, the listings are provincial, so it would be easier in most cases to look provincially for services that you may require.

UNITED STATES RESOURCES

AARP: Advocates for Older Americans

Administration on Aging (AoA): supportive home and community based services

Ageless Design: consultation services (Alzheimer's Disease)

Alzheimer's Association: supportive services

American Council of the Blind (ACB): advocates for visually impaired individuals

American Foundation for the Blind (AFB): provides services and support

American Horticultural Therapy Association (AHTA): promotes horticultural therapy

American Music Therapy Association (AMTA): promotion and resource information

American Parkinson's Disease Association (APDA): research and educational material

Meals on Wheels Association of America (MOWAA): provides food to homebound individuals

National Council on Aging (NCOA): provides information on a variety of aging services and issues.

National Senior Games Association (NSGA): promotes healthy lifestyles for older people.

National Stroke Association (NSA): provides information regarding strokes.

SeniorNet (SN): information and services to help older people become computer literate.

Young Men's Christian Association (YMCA): membership organization promoting health programs.

Young Women's Christian Association (YWCA): membership organization promoting health programs.

CANADIAN RESOURCES

Concepts du Sablier: offers products and material for people with disabilities

Spectrum Nasco Senior Activities: sells activity materials for seniors

The Division of Aging and Seniors: provides federal leadership on health issues related to aging and seniors

New Seniors Canada Site: information source for seniors

Canadian National Institute for the Blind (CNIB): programs and services for the visually impaired

Parkinson Society of Canada: provides support and education about the disease

Shoppers Drug Mart: addresses the health care needs of Canadians

The Alzheimer Society: provides support and education about the disease

The Heart and Stroke Foundation: charitable organization

GENERAL RESOURCES

Nightingale-Conant: provides audio program to help you create the life you want

Tranquilities: helps people on a path towards healing and restoration

The Sedona Method: provide support, helps to achieve balance, success, etc.

Posit Science: a brain fitness program to help people think faster, focus, and remember more

UNITED STATES

AARP

"This is a nonprofit organization that advocates for older Americans. They deal with health, rights, and life choices. Local chapters provide information and services on consumer protection, crime prevention, and income tax preparation. Members can join group health, auto, life, and home insurance programs, among other services." Publications are also available.

Address: 601 E Street NW, Washington, DC 20049

Phone 1-888-OUR-AARP (687-2277) toll-free

ADMINISTRATION ON AGING (AOA)

"The Administration on Aging works together with other agencies that are dedicated to policy development, planning, and delivery of supportive home and community based services for seniors and their caregivers."

Address: Department of Health and Human Services (DHHS), Washington, DC 20201

Telephone: Public Enquiries: 202-619-0724; Eldercare Locator: 1-800-677-1116 (toll-free)

Website: www.aoa.gov

AGELESS DESIGN

"Ageless Design offers consultation services, books, articles, audiotapes, and other resources for those caring for someone with Alzheimer's disease."

Address: 3197 Trout Place Road, Cumming, GA 30041

Telephone: 1-800-752-3238 (toll-free)

Website: www.agelessdesign.com

ALZHEIMER'S ASSOCIATION

"This association is a nonprofit organization that offers information and support to people with Alzheimer's disease and their families."

Address: 225 N. Michigan Avenue, Chicago, IL 60601

Telephone: 1-800-272-3900 (toll-free)

Website: www.alz.org

AMERICAN COUNCIL OF THE BLIND (ACB)

"ACB is a national organization that advocates for the blind and visually impaired. It provides educational programs, health care services, and other health and social services."

Address: 1155 15th Street NW, Suite 1004, Washington, DC 20005

Telephone: 1-800-424-8666 (toll-free) 202-467-5081

Website: www.acb.org

AMERICAN FOUNDATION FOR THE BLIND (AFB)

"The AFB is a national, nonprofit organization that provides services and support for people who are blind or visually impaired. They provide technologies such as the Talking Books program and along with information, books, pamphlets, videos, etc. about blindness."

Address: 11 Penn Plaza, Suite 300, New York, NY 10001

Telephone: 1-800-AFB-LINE (232-5463) (toll-free) 212-50207600

Website: www.afb.org

AMERICAN HORTICULTURAL THERAPY
ASSOCIATION (AHTA)

"The AHTA is a nonprofit organization that promotes horticultural therapy and a therapeutic intervention and rehabilitation option."

Address: 201 East Main Street, Suite 1405,
Lexington, KY 40507-2004

Telephone: 1-800-634-1603 (toll-free) 859-514-9177

Website: www.ahta.org

AMERICAN MUSIC THERAPY ASSOCIATION
(AMTA)

"The AMTA is a nonprofit organization that promotes and provides resources on the uses and benefits of music therapy."

Address: 6455 Colesville Road, Suite 1000, Silver Spring,
MD 20910

Telephone: 301-589-3300

Website: www.musictherapy.org

AMERICAN PARKINSON'S DISEASE ASSOCIATION
(APDA)

"The APDA is a nonprofit organization that funds research to find a cure for Parkinson's disease. The toll-free line refers callers to the local chapter. Publications and educational materials are available on Parkinson's disease, speech therapy, exercise, diet, and aids for daily living."

Address: 135 Parkinson Avenue, Staten Island, NY 10305

Telephone: 1-800-223-2732 (toll-free) 718-981-8001

Website: www.apdaparkinson.org

MEALS ON WHEELS ASSOCIATION OF AMERICA
(MOWAA)

"This is a national, nonprofit organization that provides training and grants to programs that provide food to older people and those who are frail or homebound."

Address: 203 S. Union Street, Alexandria, VA 22314

Telephone: 703-548-5558

Website: www.mowaa.org

NATIONAL COUNCIL ON AGING (NCOA)

"This is a private, nonprofit organization that provides information, training, advocacy, technical assistance, and leadership in all aspects of aging services and issues. They offer information on training programs and in-home services for older people. Publications are available on topics such as lifelong learning, senior center services, adult day care, long-term care, financial issues, senior housing, rural issues, intergenerational programs, and volunteers in aging."

Address: 300 D Street SW, Suite 801,
Washington, DC 20024

Telephone: 202-479-0735

Website: www.ncoa.org

NATIONAL SENIOR GAMES ASSOCIATION
(NSGA)

"The NSGA is a nonprofit organization that promotes healthy lifestyles for older people through education, fitness, and sports."

Address: P.O. Box 82059, Baton Rouge, LA 70884-2059

Telephone: 225-766-6800

Website: www.nationalseniorgames.org

RECOMMENDED RESOURCES

NATIONAL STROKE ASSOCIATION (NSA)

"The NSA provides information about stroke prevention, treatment, recovery, and rehabilitation. They offer referrals to support groups, care centers, and local resources for stroke survivors, caregivers, and family members."

Address: 9707 East Easter Lane, Building B, Englewood, CO 80127

Telephone: 1-800-STROKES (787-6537) (toll-free)

Website: www.stroke.org

SENIORNET (SN)

"SN is a nonprofit organization that provides information and services that help older people become computer literate. They offer introductory computer classes and provide older people with discounts on computer hardware, software, and publications."

Address: 900 Lafayette Street, Suite 604, Santa Clara, CA 95050

Telephone: 408-615-0699

Website: www.seniornet.org

YOUNG MEN'S CHRISTIAN ASSOCIATION (YMCA)

"This is a membership organization that provides physical fitness and other health programs. They offer an Active Older Adult program to meet the needs of older members and provide volunteer opportunities for seniors as well as offering intergenerational programs."

Address: 101 North Wacker Drive, Chicago, IL 60606

Telephone: 1-800-USA-YMCA (872-9622) (toll-free)

Website: www.ymca.net

YOUNG WOMEN'S CHRISTIAN ASSOCIATION

(YWCA)

"The YWCA is a membership organization that provides health, fitness, and community services for women. They provide education workshops, recreational activities, and counseling services."

Address: 1015 18th St. NW, Suite 1100,
Washington, DC 20036

Telephone: 1-800-YWCA-US1 (992-2871) (toll-free)
202-467-0801

Website: www.ywca.org

CANADIAN RESOURCES

CONCEPTS DU SABLIER

Concepts du Sablier offers products and materials designed for people with disabilities. "They offer a variety of 'just for fun' products as well as products for homecare therapeutic activities. Their goal is to fulfill the needs of caregivers in all environments."

Address: 2658 Galt West, Sherbrooke, QC J1K 2X2

Telephone: 1-888-907-6878

Website: www.sablier.com

SPECTRUM NASCO SENIOR ACTIVITIES

"This company provides therapeutic activities for seniors. It sells activity kits and carts, spiritual activity materials, humor books and videotapes, a variety of different games and equipment, reminiscence activity kits, and many other resources."

Address: 150 Pony Drive, Newmarket, ON L3Y 7B6

Phone: (800) 668-0600

Website: www.Spectrumed.com

THE DIVISION OF AGING AND SENIORS

"The Division of Aging and Seniors, Public Health Agency of Canada, provides federal leadership on health issues related to aging and seniors. It provides advice, encourages seniors' health promotion, and has information related to health and aging."

Address: 200 Eglantine Driveway, Ottawa, ON K1A 0K9

Phone: (613) 952-7606

Email: seniors@phac-aspc.gc.ca

NEW SENIORS CANADA SITE

"The New Seniors Canada site is Canada's premier information source for seniors, caregivers, families, and service providers."

Website: www.seniors.gc.ca

CNIB

(CANADIAN NATIONAL

INSTITUTE FOR THE BLIND)

"The CNIB provides vital programs and services, an extensive range of innovative consumer products, and one of the world's largest libraries for people with [impaired vision]."

Mail: CNIB National Office

1929 Bayview Avenue, Toronto, ON M4G 3E8

Phone: (800) 563-2642

Website: www.cnib.ca

Sales & Information Phone: (727) 803-8000 (worldwide)

Fax: (727) 803-8001

PARKINSON SOCIETY OF CANADA

"Parkinson Society Canada eases the burden of living with Parkinson's through support and education. Information and resources are available for you, your care partners, and your family members. Referrals are also made to the regional Parkinson Society for specific information on support groups, exercise programs, movement disorder clinics, and educational sessions."

Address: 4211 Yonge Street, 316, Toronto, ON M2P 2A9

Phone: (416) 227-9700

Toll-Free: (800) 565-3000

Website: www.parkinson.ca

SHOPPERS DRUG MART

"Shoppers Drug Mart has been addressing the health care needs of Canadians since 1962. The goal of their community involvement at a national and local level is to help Canadians enjoy their health and live life to the fullest. They focus on health-related programs that promote good health and prevent diseases."

Website: www.shoppersdrugmart.ca

THE ALZHEIMER SOCIETY

"The Alzheimer Society provides support, information, and education to people with Alzheimer's disease as well as their families, physicians, and health-care providers.

The Alzheimer Society arranges or refers people to support groups that provide a safe place to share information, thoughts, feelings, and experiences. They help people find programs and services they need, such as day programs and respite programs, home support, and help with the difficult transition to long-term care."

Address: 20 Eglinton Avenue W., Suite 1200,
Toronto, ON M4R 1K8

Telephone: (416) 488-8772

Toll-free: (800) 616-8816 (valid only in Canada)

Website: www.alzheimer.ca

THE HEART AND STROKE FOUNDATION

"The Heart and Stroke Foundation is a volunteer-based health charity organization."

Address: 222 Queen Street, Suite 1402,
Ottawa, ON K1P 5V9

Telephone: (613) 569-4361

Website: www.heartandstroke.com

GENERAL RECOMMENDED RESOURCES

NIGHTINGALE-CONANT

Audio programs and customized resources to help you create the life you want.

Telephone: (800) 557-1660

Nightingale-Conant

6245 W. Howard Street, Niles, IL 60714

Website: www.nightingale.com

TRANQUILITIES

Emotional and spiritual support for life's challenges

http://www.tranquilities.com/

GILEAD ENTERPRISES

"Gilead Enterprises, Inc. (Gilead) was formed in 2002 to provide innovative products to provide spiritual and emotional support for individuals dealing with stressful life situations. Located in northern Lancaster County, Pennsylvania, the company was birthed when the Ephrata Community Hospital commissioned its Mind, Body and Spirit task force to create a guided imagery program for patients."

247 North Reading Road

Ephrata, PA 17522

Phone: (717) 721-6998

Website: www.gileadenterprises.com

THE SEDONA METHOD

"Transforming Minds—Transforming Lives Worldwide Through the Sedona Method and the Holistic Releasing Process. Their mission is to be supportive in alleviating physical and emotional suffering and liberating natural inner freedom to have, be, and do whatever your heart desires. They also support individuals and organizations in achieving balance, success, wellness, strength, effectiveness, happiness, and well-being. Their goal and mission is to help people all over the world to free themselves of limiting thoughts, feelings, and behaviors so they can live the lives they want—having, being, and doing whatever their heart desires, and thereby achieving their full potential."

Address: 60 Tortilla Drive, Sedona, AZ 86336

Toll-Free: (888) 282-5656

Phone: (928) 282-3522

Website: www.sedona.com

POSIT SCIENCE

THE BRAIN FITNESS PROGRAM CLASSIC

"The Brain Fitness Program is a computer-based software program clinically proven to help people think faster, focus better, and remember more."

Address: 225 Bush Street, Seventh Floor,
San Francisco, CA 94104

Phone: (800) 514-3961

Website: www.positscience.com

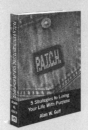
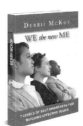
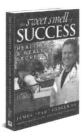
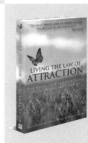
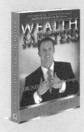
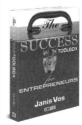
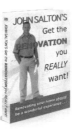
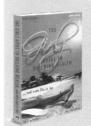

Other books from **LifeSuccess PUBLISHING**

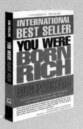

You Were Born Rich

Bob Proctor

ISBN 978-0-9656264-1-5

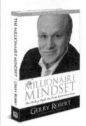

The Millionaire Mindset

How Ordinary People Can Create Extraordinary Income

Gerry Robert

ISBN 978-1-59930-030-6

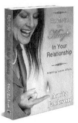

Rekindle The Magic In Your Relationship

Making Love Work

Anita Jackson

ISBN 978-1-59930-041-2

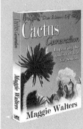

Finding The Bloom of The Cactus Generation

Improving the quality of life for Seniors

Maggie Walters

ISBN 978-1-59930-011-5

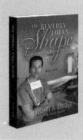

The Beverly Hills Shape

The Truth About Plastic Surgery

Dr. Stuart Linder

ISBN 978-1-59930-049-8

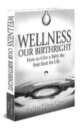

Wellness Our Birthright

How to give a baby the best start in life.

Vivien Clere Green

ISBN 978-1-59930-020-7

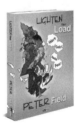

Lighten Your Load

Peter Field

ISBN 978-1-59930-000-9

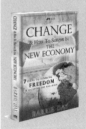

Change & How To Survive In The New Economy

7 steps to finding freedom & escaping the rat race

Barrie Day

ISBN 978-1-59930-015-3

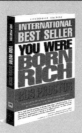
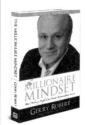
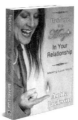
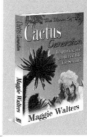
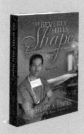
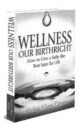
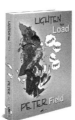
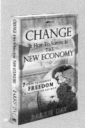

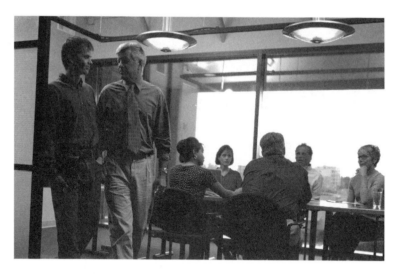

SHARE THIS MESSAGE

Bulk Discounts
Discounts start at a low number of copies, ranging from 30% to 50% off based on the quantity chosen.

Custom Publishing
Would you like a private label or a customization to suit your needs? We could even highlight specific chapters.

Sponsorship
Would you like to sponsor this book? It's a great way to advertise your product or service in a unique way!

Dynamic Speakers
Authors are available to you, to share their expertise at your event!

Call LifeSuccess Publishing at 1-800-473-7134 or email
info@lifesuccesspublishing.com for more information

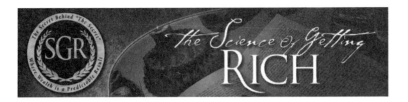

The Secret Behind *"The Secret"*

THE SCIENCE OF GETTING RICH

Home Study Course: *$1,995.00*

More Powerful than Any DVD, Book, Seminar or Course!

Here's What You Will Get...

1. Never-Before-Recorded Audio Instruction

With this program, you will be one of the privileged few to get access to never-before-recorded audio instruction and summaries of lessons and observations from the Teachers Bob Proctor and Jack Canfield. This is 10 audio CDs jam packed with their tutelage.

2. Bob Proctor and Jack Canfield, always by your side.

We will also give you a compact digital MP3 player pre-loaded with 15-hours of content which means you will be totally immersed in the program IMMEDIATELY and CONSTANTLY to ensure you effect the Law of Attraction to bring you wealth EVERYDAY!

Immerse yourself anytime and anywhere! Listen anytime while in a bus, on a train, waiting in line, during lunch breaks, by the pool...

3. Tools To Help You Take Action and Keep It Going

15 Dynamic Lessons that capture specific teachings to help you further understand and implement the Law of Attraction as well as other Universal Laws. Clearly taught by Bob Proctor and Summarized by Jack Canfield.

Compact Personal Vision Boards for mapping out and envisioning the life you seek to attract.

Multiple Sources of Income (MSI) Whiteboards that motivate and inspire you to create New Channels of Wealth.

A Science of Getting Rich Goal Card - one of the primary foundational pieces in the absolute realization of your dreams.

4. New Opportunities, A Support System, Continuous Learning

$500 Gift Certificate to attend a live seminar worldwide to continue learning in a live seminar environment!

Instant and Global Connections for all your networking and connection needs. It's online, active communities, masterminds, blogs and discussion boards that welcome your participation and insights as you grow through this tremendous process.

The Original Science of Getting Rich Book beautifully redesigned for this Briefcase, which means that ANYONE can master and internalize the wisdom of the ORIGINAL text without exception!

5. A Complete Training System in One Powerful Briefcase

A Rich, Supple Leather-Bound Briefcase specially designed to contain The Home Seminar Kit so that you can take it with you EVERYWHERE with no hassle. ALL THIS Delivered to your doorstep.

ORDER YOUR BRIEFCASE TODAY AT:
www.sgroilmd.com